Dedication

To my wonderful and truly amazing husband Len.

Words alone cannot express how much I love and appreciate

you. When I met and married you,

I had no idea what a perfect choice you were for me.

God knew!

I love you. Now and forever. xx

Diamonds in the Dark

Diamonds in the Dark

How One Woman's Faith Carried Her Through
Two Diagnoses of Cancer

Heather Magee

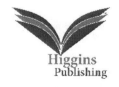

Higgins
Publishing

All scripture quotations, unless otherwise indicated, are taken from The HOLY BIBLE, New International Version®. NIV ® Copyright © 2011, by Biblica, Inc.™ Used by permission of Zondervan. All rights reserved worldwide. www.zondervan.com The "NIV" and "New International Version" are trademarks registered in the United States Patent and Trademark Office by Biblica, Inc. Other translations used and noted where appropriate:

Published by Higgins Publishing
1.877.788.5613 | www.higginspublishing.com

Higgins Publishing is committed to excellence in the publishing industry. The company reflects the philosophy established by the founder, based on Psalm 68:11,
"The Lord gave the word, and great was the company of those who published it."

Book & Cover design Copyright © 2016-2017 by Higgins Publishing. All Rights Reserved.

The Higgins Publishing Speakers Bureau provides a wide range of authors for speaking events. To schedule an author for an event, go to www.higginspublishing.com.

Library of Congress Cataloging-in-Publication Data
Magee, Heather
Diamonds in the Dark – Heather Magee – First Higgins Publishing softcover edition – October 2017
      pages cm. 316
ISBN: 978-1-941580-14-1 (sc)   Control Number: 2016930438

1.   Christian Life: General
2.   Christian Life: Women's Issues
3.   Christian Life: Spiritual Warfare

For information about special discounts for bulk purchases, subsidiary, foreign and translations rights & permissions, please contact Higgins Publishing at 1.877.788.5613 or business@higginspublishing.com * Published in the United States of America.

TABLE OF CONTENTS

Foreword

I count it a huge privilege to be asked to write a foreword for this book and to be invited into the vulnerable pages of this season of Heather's journey. She has taken us to the depths of human suffering, with all its sickness, trauma, doubts, and fears.

Many who read these pages will truly relate to the authenticity of the physical and emotional suffering that Heather so honestly describes. However, she's not left us there to languish in its dreaded clutches. She offers us heartfelt answers and a genuinely balanced theology for suffering, from both a human and God perspective. I found this book riveting in its content. Writing with transparency and from a pure heart, she portrays a picture that will both inspire and encourage weary, suffering travelers and give them new hope for their future.

This is more than a book. It really is a life map to guide those on a similar path and learn from its ruthlessly honest pages; how to cope, where to turn in trouble, and how to remain steadfast when going through life's valley experiences. I commend this book very highly, from one who has also traveled the journey and found God's grace in every situation.

Dr. Ray Andrews

"Shortly after the recent floods, I was driving across central Queensland. The road was badly damaged by the heavy deluges and we were forced to travel slowly. A flashing sign on the side of the road caught my attention and totally transformed the journey. It said, 'Ignore your GPS! There is a better road ahead!' Heather has chosen to ignore the natural GPS of looking at her circumstances and has fixed her eyes on Jesus for the better road He has marked out for her. This is the amazing story of Heather's determination to persevere through her many trials and trust God in all things. Parts brought me to tears as I learned of her journey, and parts reaffirmed my trust in the God who created us and loves us perfectly. Heather, thanks for the privilege of reading your story!"

Joan Pennicook (Wife of Pastor John Pennicook)

Introduction

I love real-life stories. Whenever Len and I go away for a mini break, I head straight to the bookshop and sift through the biography section until I find a story that looks captivating. Then during the next few days, I'll lose myself in someone else's life experience. Great diversional therapy!

Some stories though, are devastating. We are constantly being bombarded by powerful images attached to carefully written scripts, as journalists push our minds past realistic boundaries. Reports of daily disasters tug at our heartstrings, as they portray emotions that become increasingly hard to process.

I remember the time when terrorists attacked London. Images were flashed around the world, showing a young woman bleeding, crying out for her lost boyfriend. We saw a fireman patching her up before she was hurried away in an ambulance and disappeared from view. What happened to her? Did she survive the blast? We were left wondering.

Right now, you are in the middle a story. God is writing it and you are living it. However, our stories are real-life dramas, not just fantasy Hollywood novels. Everyone's experience is unique. Like snowflakes, no two are ever the same. But we all have one thing in common. In some way and at some time, we will suffer. Just a few scenarios come to mind:

- The mother who pulled her 3-year-old baby lifeless from a swimming pool.

- The woman who lost her first baby, just 6 hours after he was born.

- A young girl watching her father and grandfather build war shelters in their garden, fearing that at any moment a bomb might fall and obliterate her whole family.

- A small child fostered out from her family for safety, when bombs dropped on London during the war. Would she ever see her mum and dad again? Fear and insecurity became her unwelcome companions.

- The six-year-old boy given away by his mother and sent on a ship across the world because she couldn't look after him. An abusive institution became the oppressive backdrop for the start of his young life.

- The unexpected phone call that startles a young wife saying, "Your husband is dangerously ill in hospital, and we're not sure if he will survive."

- Disease, accidents and trauma that dramatically change your life forever; both for you and every other family member.

- A sickness that comes out of the blue, completely left-field, that no specialist can diagnose or knows how to treat, which brings years of loss and tragic deprivation.

- A baby abandoned at birth, adopted by cruel parents and treated like a slave. She lived behind walls of a secret prison.

➤ The stroke that suddenly leaves a loved one unable to walk or talk, unsure of the prognosis for the rest of his life.

➤ Times of stunning betrayal, loneliness, misunderstandings, loss and grief.

These are just excerpts from the journals of my own extended family. Yet over the years, I've heard other people's stories that have left me dumbfounded.

One was of a Jewish woman who fell in love with a man she later discovered was anti-Semitic. After he'd tried to kill her several times, she extricated herself from his evil grasp. Scraping up the few fragments left from her wretched relationship, she escaped with her small children. Hopelessness and despair wrought absolute havoc in the lives of this little family.

I remember talking with another woman, whose ex-husband had hung himself above the altar of a Catholic Cathedral. He was found by a very surprised priest! How could I begin to relate to her? I simply listened amazed, trying to imagine her pain and understand her confusion. It was mind blowing!

Everyone's journeys are different and so are our experiences. There are no safe guarantees that everything will be amazing on this pilgrimage called 'Life!' Some may be attacked by proverbial wild lions. (Hopefully not!) Others may fall down cleverly camouflaged potholes. Those seemingly more fortunate, might go straight to the top of the mountain, without many dramas at all. Excellent health, thriving businesses, perfect partners, loving families, beautiful kids who always do as they're told (don't know many of those however), and understanding friends who are there when you need them at the slightest call.

Even today, while writing this introduction, I watched a few minutes of a chat show on the TV. It was Australia Day. A woman who was a billionaire was being interviewed. Sitting beside her was her sister, expressing that in her opinion, her rich sister was the worst parent she knew, because she threw $1 million parties for her kids and gave them everything they wanted. Unfortunately, that also included things they didn't want, such as bodyguards who followed them constantly! Oh, the vitriol and jealousy that was expressed for all to see. How sad. Even the wealthy have their problems. Money is certainly no guarantee that everyone will love you; neither does it mean you will always be deliriously happy.

Each situation in life has its own possibilities for potential pain and misunderstanding. Some come with inbuilt challenges that can leave you breathless at times! I'm sure you could also give your own accounts; some heart-breaking, some inspiring and courageous, and some unbelievably miraculous.

This book you are reading is just part of my story, my journey with cancer. Never did I imagine that I would ever write about such an experience; but then, you may have gone through far worse than I have. Nevertheless, who's comparing which experiences are more desperate or dramatic in their detail? I feel it's not so much what we go through, but how we walk through our individual circumstances that is important. What we learn can be life changing and the fact that we eventually come out into the light at the end of the tunnel is what really matters.

I am just praying that you will be able to relate to some of my experiences and that as you read these pages, we can join our hands and our hearts together for a short while. I hope that you will draw some encouragement from some of the lessons I have learned along the way.

~~

A few years ago, I wrote this poem and filed it in my notebook. It was after we had moved interstate. We'd said goodbye to some very dear friends and were being replanted in a new location. I was aware we were entering a new season, but wasn't quite sure what to expect. The change wasn't easy. Everything was new and different. Once again, I was learning new levels of trust.

I cannot see around the corner
If there are seas of stormy water
Or glassy streams that wend their ways
Through hazy glow of summer days.
It could be that dark clouds arise
Obscuring sunlight from my eyes,
Or it might be that new spring rains
Will fall, refreshing barren plains.

I do not know, but one thing's sure
It's God who plans my way; and more
And more as time goes by
I'll understand the reasons why
The seasons of my life must change
And some things will be rearranged.
But He's the One who knows me best
And in that knowledge, I can rest.

For He wants me to believe
That everything He does for me
Is from my Father's loving hand,
To bring to pass the things He's planned.
So, though I can't see with my eyes
The coming weather in the skies,
I'll trust the One whose Word is true
To walk with me and bring me through!

Little did I realize that these words penned previously would have such great significance, so many years later!

Section A
My Story

CHAPTER ONE

Never Would I Have Imagined!

Some birthdays are more momentous than others. The one that stands out for me is the celebration we had for my 50th. It was such a special occasion. Friends and family (my mum and dad were still alive at this time) gathered around to share their love with me, and to this day I remember how deeply it touched my heart. That night on the way home, many memories came flooding back. Where had the last five decades gone?

At the age of 25, I had emigrated from England to Australia with my husband Len, leaving behind all my family and childhood friends. My mum and dad had wept with us when we told them we were going to co-pastor a church in Australia (where my husband had grown up as a child migrant). It was only a few months and we were gone, leaving to serve the Lord in a country I didn't know, with people I'd never met. At that time, I hadn't even learned to drive! So while Len was at work, I was at home with an 18-month old toddler. I had no parents or grandparents to call on, no sisters to share in my world, and my dearest friends were back home on the other side of the globe!

It was however, an amazing time in my life. I knew without a doubt that I was perfectly placed in the will of God. Sure, I wept when we boarded the plane, having said our final goodbyes. I cried for six hours. I felt my heart was literally going to break. Strangely though, my emotions were tinged with a strange color of joy. Little did I know that this would become a familiar feeling through many of the unimagined sorrows I would experience.

Life in the ministry was always going to be a challenge. That became apparent from day one! However, I was married to the man of my dreams; a well-known gospel singer and songwriter, who 'just happened' to have been called by God to preach His Word. I could not have written the script for my life any better myself. The heady days of our courtship had been more romantic than I had certainly ever dreamed.

Nine months later we were married (no significance in that by the way!) and committed ourselves to each other; 'For better and for worse, for richer, for poorer, till death do us part.' United we stood, earnest in our love for the Lord and each other. Bulletproof and invincible. (So we thought!)

Our lives collided in marriage. 'Collided' being the operative word, because that's what happens when two streams from entirely different directions meet and merge into one major river. There was a lot of white water rafting as the tumbling waters converged, but it was fun. We learned to laugh, forgive and pray our way through our first few years. (We still do!) We were with each other, and that was all that mattered. I knew the Lord had brought us together. We were in love. I would have followed my husband anywhere in the world. And so I did.

However, like many others, I would face some dark times and harsh realities of pressure and pain. I didn't know God had such an agenda for me, this side of eternity. (That was His secret!) Neither did I realize that God was in the divine 'jewelry business' fashioning precious stones, and what a process it was going to be as He worked on me!

Diamonds

A diamond is a precious stone made from crystalized carbon, a highly valuable gem, far rarer than gold. It has been estimated that up to 183,600 tons of gold have been mined throughout the world, compared to only 500 tons of diamonds. (Rare indeed!) Where do diamonds originate? Well, they don't grow on trees unfortunately, otherwise I would be growing a few in my back yard! Most of them are buried deep in the dirt somewhere, remaining hidden and of no monetary value until they are eventually discovered.

Sadly, diamonds don't suddenly pop to the surface of the soil, ready to wear! They are mined from darkness, where they have been buried for thousands of years. Unlike other stones that are formed in the earth's crust, diamonds are forged in the deep underground layer of volcanic magna called the mantle, where temperatures can reach up to 1,000 degrees centigrade.

The pressure at such depths is more than is physically possible to endure. (No one has dived down to the ocean floor and survived without wearing protective equipment.) Nevertheless, that is only one-fiftieth of the compression found in the volcanic mantle where these treasures are made! What immense and continuous exertion of force! But, look what it produces – diamonds that are tough and endurable, brilliant and beautiful. And extremely valuable!

There are probably billions of undiscovered diamonds that we walk on unknowingly, because they are concealed so far below the earth's surface. (So sad!) However, those that reach the surface are usually deposited there by massive underground explosions. These are known as 'kimberlite pipes' which fire the magna to the face of the earth at speeds of up to 180 mph! Yet, not all the volcanic pipes carry the coveted crystals. Only 1 in every 200 contain the diamond gems. (So scarce!)

After the jewels have been lifted to ground level, they can then be fossicked for and gratefully found. But, they have to go through many various stages of being shaped and skillfully fashioned, before their true beauty is seen. What a procedure this is!

The diamond must be cut. Did I say the word 'cut'? Oh no! Incredible amounts of patience and skill are required to transform one of the world's hardest natural materials into a highly polished precious stone. The ultimate goal of a diamond cutter is to produce the best cut and most carat weight out of the raw material he has to work with. The diamond is meticulously placed, ready for sawing. Did I say sawing? Yes! A circular diamond-coated saw will divide this rough gem into separate pieces. Each one has to be cut precisely and appropriately, with the greatest sensitivity, allowing for their unique individual differences.

Then comes the 'bruting' process. Two diamonds are set onto spinning axles turning in completely opposite directions, which are positioned purposely to grind against each other as they are shaped and rounded out. Maybe this is part of God's purpose in marriage! One diamond thrust against the other. Bruting sounds about right!

The final stage of the cutting process and most crucial is called 'blocking.' This determines the diamond's fundamental symmetry. It may not seem significant, but it is. Just minor inconsistencies in symmetry and proportions can make all the difference between a gorgeous diamond and a dull, lifeless stone. This process is essential for giving the diamond its greatest potential. Between seventeen to fifty-eight facets are carefully cut to refract the fire of color that will eventually radiate from inside the jewel.

The larger diamonds are then sent away for the 'brillianteering' stage where the final facets are polished. Not more friction? Yes, because the more rubbing and buffing a diamond endures, the more brilliance it will ultimately display. However, before the last critical inspection, they are also cleaned in acids! Now they glisten!

But, I want to be all brilliant and beautiful now! Yes of course I want to shine and reflect flashes of radiant color, displaying God's glory in my life. Nevertheless, will I yield to the cutting saw, and the rubbing together with the other rough diamonds? Can I endure the bruting and the buffing that is so necessary to create the sparkle? If I'm to be one of God's gems, then I must expect the Designer's use of the sharp blades! I didn't know it would be so literal!

I am aware that even now, you may be going through intense pressure, more than I have, or perhaps ever will experience. But it's all going to be worth it. The value God places on us is priceless.

And the end result is going to be spectacular!

CHAPTER TWO

The Beginning of One Unpredictable Journey

No one could have prepared me for the emotions that I would experience as I entered my fifth decade. Wasn't life meant to begin at fifty? At least, that's what they told me! So I was ready to enjoy this new season with renewed anticipation and drink every drop of nectar that I could possibly squeeze out of it. However, my sister Libby sowed a seed thought over one of our regular cups of coffee. "Heather, you've just turned fifty. It's about time you had a 'grease and oil change'. When was your last mammogram?" To be honest, I hadn't even given it a second thought. Having cancer was not on my 'to-do' list. It had never entered my imagination. But the thought persisted. Perhaps I should at least check. So casually, I booked an appointment.

Therefore, when the receptionist from the breast clinic called me to say that my X-ray had shown up some strange imaging, and asked me to return, I remember feeling rather blasé. Maybe they had rung the wrong number. They were surely looking for someone else. When I expressed my surprise, a kind-hearted woman assured me that their call was only routine, and in a situation like this I need not be at all concerned.

So, it *was* me they were trying to contact! Oh no! What could be wrong? My stress immediately rocketed to undiscovered heights. Generally, I have a philosophy not to worry until there is something to worry about and then pray like the clappers! This time though, it was easier said than done!

Two short days seemed like two long weeks. I hoped they had made a mistake. I tried to bury my trepidation and hide the anxiety that threatened to overwhelm me, but my nerves were taut and felt ready to snap. Nevertheless, by the time the appointment eventually came, I had convinced myself that this was just going to be a quick routine check. I hopped in my car, quite sure I would be home in less than an hour, with the news that all was well.

Seven hours later, I was still at the clinic! What was happening to me? Why did they keep sending me from one room to the other, for further investigations and more tests? They started by repeating my mammogram. Well, I expected that. Then they sent me back to the waiting room where you do just that! WAIT! I think I read an out-of-date women's magazine to fill my mind up with anything except the case at hand. I was sure that they would release me in a few more minutes with the news that all was fine and I could go home. But, minutes turned into segments of half hours. Now they were insisting I needed an ultrasound. Suddenly, this was becoming a lot more serious than I had expected. Oh well, at least ultrasounds don't hurt. It would be over soon.

There was one disturbing fact. One nurse was suddenly joined by two other nurses. Together, they looked grimly at the images on the screen above me. What were they all inspecting so inquisitively? Whatever it was, they kept surprisingly quiet, as though they were guarding a private secret. Why wouldn't they tell me? Suspicious thoughts seeped into my heart like toxic poison. Once again, I was sent back to the waiting room. The women's magazines were no longer able to desensitize my mind and silence my internal screams. Fortunately, no one could hear but then, no one seemed to care anyway. I remained alone with my tumble-dryer of emotions for what seemed like an eternity.

As my mind battled bewilderment, someone called my name. "Heather, come this way. We need to do a bilateral biopsy!" Surely not! I knew the word biopsy! It was synonymous with pain. Oh no! I assumed they'd give me some sort of anesthetic so I wouldn't feel anything. Well, I won't go into the details here but, needless to say, I was not prepared for the type of procedure I was about to endure.

The nurses were lovely and tried to reassure me with kind words but I really wasn't listening. All I knew was the positive way my day had started, was not how it was about to finish. I just wanted to be home with my husband and do what the English do after a difficult day. Have a good cup of tea!

However, I wasn't at home. I was incarcerated in the breast clinic. Now I was extremely sore and swelling fast. Everyone else appeared to have left, but here I was, lying on a clinical bed with a concerned nurse talking about the fact that I might have to go to hospital. I was quickly turning multiple shades of black and blue. I think they had accidentally hit an artery, so it looked likely I would need further treatment.

My recollection of the next few minutes is rather hazy. My eyes began to leak and my heart was bursting with fear. Wasn't I meant to be full of faith? After all, I was a pastor's wife and had comforted many in their fiery furnaces. Now I was in one of my own, and the fire just seemed to be getting hotter by the second. At least in the biblical story of Shadrach, Meshach and Abednego, they were in the furnace together (Daniel 3:21-23). I was just left in the room alone with my frightened feelings.

Thoughts swarmed around me like a cacophony of screaming vultures, with no one to shoo them away. What were they going to do with me? Apparently, not very much at all. They finally stopped the incessant blood flow with a compressed ice pack. I could leave at last. I gathered up my confusion with my belongings, and walked out of the clinic. I was going home but not in the same buoyant way I had left. I was glad I'd soon find solace in the arms of my husband. How would he process all this? I couldn't even begin to untangle my thoughts. What are you supposed to feel in moments like these?

He was amazing! His loving arms wrapped snuggly around me the moment I fell in the door. Holding me tight, he whispered, "It'll be alright darling, you'll see! We'll walk through this together. The Lord is sovereign. He has promised to work all things together for good. Let's watch Him work and see what He will do. I love you, and nothing will change that. If the tests come back and show you have breast cancer, we'll face the consequences then. For now, we'll roll this burden on the Lord. He will sustain us."

The trouble was that I would have to wait the whole weekend until I'd know the results. Trust me, these few days felt like forever. Only my closest friends and family knew of my ordeal. Len still preached and I led the worship. We continued living as normal and for us, that meant being with our loving church family and praising the Lord 'whatever.'

As one might expect, daunting thoughts that I could actually die did dart across my mind, but that didn't mean God had changed. He remained worthy of my love and praise. After all, if I was going to meet Him sooner than I had planned, then I'd better be prepared!

At that time, I was faced with an important choice. The saying, "It's not what you have to deal with that is the issue, it's how you walk through it that counts," was never more significant to me than

31

in this situation. Each day is a day that the Lord has made. We can choose to believe God's promise to work all things together for our good according to His purposes, or we can despair and be miserable making everyone else depressed as well! I know which I'd prefer.

George Muller (well known for his incredible faith and who I will mention again later), once gave this testimony; "It is possible, and I am proof. I have rolled my burdens on the Lord and He has carried them for me. The result of that has been 'the peace of God which passes all understanding' which has kept my heart and mind. For more than seventy years I have not been anxious."

What an amazing statement from this spiritual giant. To pass the examination of trust at this level, I am well aware I have many more experiences to go through, and many more lessons to learn! Although, nothing could have fully prepared me for my next few semesters!

CHAPTER THREE

The Pit of Despair

I have discovered that fear and anxiety are like twin potholes, well positioned to fall into if you're not looking, with little help available when you are sick of the misery, and you want to get out. I distinctly recall an event that happened many years ago, when I first fell right into the trap.

Our 9-year-old son Matthew developed a mystery illness. He came home from school happy and healthy, but the next morning as he tried to get out of bed, he could hardly move. He was almost paralyzed with weakness. During the following days, overwhelming fatigue set in like a rainy season in the tropics, with no end in sight. Day after day he languished until he no longer even had the strength to lift his fork and feed himself. This debilitating condition persisted for three long months No doctors could give me any idea as to what was the cause. Recommendations were even made to test him for Polio and Guillain-Barre Syndrome. I hadn't braced for this! Before long, I started to taste the sickening flavors of fear and panic. This was my boy. Mothers were supposed to fix things and make them better. They were meant to make bad things good again. But what could I do?

Well, I prayed to God with all my heart. Every day, Len and I asked for a miracle. We shared the situation with our church family. They gathered around in loving concern as perplexed as we all were, wishing they could do something – anything to make things better. The leaders in our church came to our house and prayed for Matt. By this time, I was desperate.

I believed in healing and I still do to this day, so why was Matt still sick? Hadn't God heard our urgent cries? I knew He had the power, so what was causing the blockage? Didn't the Lord want to do a miracle so that we could tell everyone how good He was? What would our congregation think? We were their pastors! We preached about miracles and faith. Surely, this was the perfect opportunity for God to demonstrate His loving kindness, so we could testify to answered prayer…wasn't it?

Before long, I had fallen headlong into the pit of despair and began nibbling on the stale bread of bitterness. I remember leading worship in our church one Sunday morning, and it was all I could do to fight back the tears. My mind told me that God was good, but my heart could not feel it. If God was so good, why did Matt have to suffer such an endless, seemingly pointless illness that no doctor could diagnose and no medical test could pinpoint?

I believed that Matt would be healed and everything would be okay, but it wasn't. If anything, his condition became worse. Surely, things weren't meant to happen this way! Len and I had prayed for numerous people in church. Many later testified to experiencing His healing power. So why wouldn't the Lord answer our requests for help, when asking for our own son to be healed?

I had it all worked out. If I were God, I would take advantage of this situation and use it to display my powers. It would hopefully impress the neighbors and be a great encouragement to the church! But, I am not God, neither do I understand His eternal purposes or have access to His unsearchable wisdom. Oh, I had (and still have) so much to learn!

The next plan of action was to gather as many pastors we knew who had well-respected healing ministries and ask them to pray for Matt. (It's strange how we can think it's more effective when others pray.) Willingly they came and fervently they prayed; so we waited with renewed faith and anticipation, believing to see the miracle we longed for.

Days merged hazily into weeks. Then weeks spilled over into months, with still no end in sight. Valuable schoolwork was missed. Matt was becoming more depressed and frustrated. A syrupy voice began to speak into my mind, "If God loves you and cares so much, why is He not listening to you? After all, you are serving Him, and telling everyone how good He is. How could God let this happen? Would you do this to someone you loved? How can you still have faith when nothing is happening? What are people going to think of your ministry now?"

On and on the insinuations battered my heart. I was struggling to stand against a plethora of fiery darts. Some penetrated their way deep into my heart. If only there were an antiseptic that could have disinfected the painful inflammation that was spreading in my soul. My faith was being stretched to the limit, like a violin string being tightly wound to its full extension, before finally reaching breaking point!

As time dragged on, it wasn't long before I became angry with everyone. I began snapping at Len and became ungracious at home. At times, I feared going to church. I didn't want anyone to see my vulnerability and tears. I was there to encourage others in their faith. Now mine was in need of repair!

I was utterly entrenched in the 'pit of despair,' or 'the slough of despond' that John Bunyan so aptly portrays in *Pilgrim's Progress*. Whilst imprisoned in a dark and dismal dungeon (accused of being an unlawful and zealous preacher in the seventeenth century), he wrote the well-known classic that has been hailed as a masterpiece. In the first chapter, he describes Christian's journey to the 'Celestial City' (heaven) and vividly depicts a scene I was experiencing so well:

Christian had a friend called Pliable. Together, they set out on an expedition, with great hopes of reaching their destination. But it wasn't long before they came across a marshy swamp in the middle of a field. The name of this slough was "Despond." Unfortunately, they didn't see it in time, before both of them were soon bathing in a slimy pool of mud. Christian was carrying such a heavy backpack, that he quickly began to sink down into the mire.

Pliable was clearly unimpressed. What were they going to do? He had only been persuaded to join with Christian because the City where they were going sounded so amazing. Now here they were, stuck in a bog! He was livid and vented his frustrations to his fellow traveler:

"Is this the happiness you told me about? If we have this much trouble after just setting out, what may we expect between now and the end of our journey?" Such was his fury, that he vowed if he ever made it out alive, he was going straight back home. Christian could continue, all by himself.

After an exhausting struggle, Pliable eventually pulled himself out of the quagmire, leaving his friend to wallow in the sludge alone. Christian tried to make his way to the other side and scramble out, but the heavy burden on his back made his frantic grasp for freedom seem impossible.

Just then, a man called 'Help' passed by and kindly offered to pull Christian out, which he did! Back on solid ground again! How good that felt! 'Help' then explained to him about the pit he had unwarily fallen into. It was named the 'Slough of Despond' because it was such a bleak and depressing place; a prolific breeding ground for many doubts and fears that lay in wait like quicksand for the unsuspecting traveler.

Fortunately, there were some sturdy steps in the middle of the slough! However, these life-saving ladders usually remained hidden because of the filth that flowed into the pit. They were disguised so well, that those who fell into the mire could not always see them, let alone find them! Consequently, many were never able to escape from their dire predicaments and so stayed bogged down in their misery and despair...even though the steps were positioned there all the time!

~~

Well, that was a perfect picture of how I was feeling. In my confusion and sorrow, I hadn't seen the pit I had fallen into, and I certainly hadn't seen the steps camouflaged against my murky soul. How depressing it was down there. I had never felt so desolate. I didn't want to talk to anyone, not even God. And it appeared that He wasn't helping anyway. So I cut off my lifelines, one by one.

The trouble was, now I was down a dark, stinking hole, all on my own, with no one to get me out. There I stayed, for as long as it took me to realize that I *never* wanted to go there again! Thank God, He sent a man called 'Help' to throw down a lifeline for me. Ken, a pastor friend of ours, rang our house one day and I took the call. I can't even remember why he rang, but I think he wanted to speak with Len, who wasn't home at the time. In the course of our conversation, he asked me the question (which has been asked a thousand times since), "How's Matt?" I probably didn't answer in the most gracious way, but I knew him well enough to be bluntly honest, so off I went on a tirade about how Matt was and how angry I was with the whole situation, including God.

Graciously, Ken let me ramble on until I had exhausted all my complaints and frustrations. Then he answered. (A great counseling tip, by the way!)

"Heather! If there's one thing I would say to you, it's this. Do you remember Job in the Old Testament and all he went through? The losses of his children, his cattle, and his health. The impact on him was indescribable. However, his wife remained…for better or for worse! A great help she definitely was not! Surely, this was the time when Job needed her most, with a word of encouragement, a gentle touch, and some loving understanding when he felt so weak. Sadly, what Job experienced was exactly the opposite! Curtly she counselled, 'Why not just curse God and die?' (So caring!) What Job needed and what he received were two entirely different things!"

Ken concluded, "Heather, that is just what the enemy of your soul wants you to do; he wants you to be angry with God, he wants you to blame Him, he wants you to become bitter and doubt God's love. Then he can still your joy and slam you mercilessly inside the dungeon of despair. However, God is the One who loves you most. He will never leave you. He is with you right now to help you.

Nevertheless, if you cut the lifeline of trust in His love, you will feel very alone."

That was exactly how I had been feeling! Job's answer to his wife is interesting. With all that he'd been through, you would have thought he may have agreed with her. He didn't at all, but he posed a great question. "Shall we accept good from God and not trouble?" The Bible tells us that in all of this, he did not sin with his mouth. He was one amazing man.

Ken reminded me that Job did not have any idea about the spiritual battle going on in the heavenly realm. He had no idea how wonderfully God was going to bless him in the latter part of his life. Yet, even though it appeared that Job's life had become a seemingly endless disaster and he couldn't see the future, his heart remained firmly steadfast, as he trusted in God. Incredibly his response was, "though He slay me, yet will I trust in Him" (Job 13:15 KJV).

Little did I know how significant this verse would be to me in the coming years. This was the most incredible revelation. It was as if the Lord had taken a heavenly torch light and shone it right into my despondant heart. I thanked Ken for his counsel, said goodbye, and then immediately dropped to my knees on the kitchen floor. I was deeply smitten.

Thankfully, I was on my own. I told the Lord how sorry I was for my complaints and dwindling faith in His goodness, whatever my circumstances were. I certainly did not want to end up like Job's wife and be a misery to everyone. I longed to draw close to God and renew my trust in Him. At that moment, I climbed the steps of my own 'slough of despond.' I hadn't seen they had been there all the time! How good it was to feel the warmth of God's love again. Help had come, and the Lord filled my heart with joy. He lifted me out of my 'pit of despair.'

The Psalmist had been there too! He had experienced slipping and sliding in the miry clay. Many were the times he despaired for his life. He had sunk down in the absence of comfort and support, before discovering the foothold of divine help. God hadn't left him to struggle alone, but had reached down, lifted him out of his misery and placed his feet on solid ground. No wonder David overflowed with gratitude…

"I waited patiently for the Lord to help me,
     and He turned to me and heard my cry.
He lifted me out of the slimy pit,
     out of the mud and mire.
He set my feet on solid ground
     and steadied me as I walked along.
He has given me a new song to sing,
     a hymn of praise to our God.
Many will see what He has done and be astounded.
     They will put their trust in the Lord
Oh, the joys of those who trust the Lord…"

(Psalm 40:1-4 NLT)

That was what I longed for more than anything. To feel a new song bubbling up in my heart. How good it felt to be back in a close relationship with the Lord and sense His presence once again. Faith began to spring up in my heart. No longer did I feel so desolate and alone.

Interestingly, it was soon after my change of heart, that Matt's miracle came. One day, he stood up with renewed strength and the following day returned to school. Oh, the relief, the lightness in my spirit, the thanks to God for hearing our desperation and answering our cries. As Job said in the midst of his trials,

"But He knows the way that I take;

When He has tried me, I shall come forth as gold" (Job 23:10 NASB).

If only I'd been able to say those words in the night season of our trial, I would have saved myself so much pain. I'd read the verse before, but it had never become as meaningful to me as it did then. I prayed, "Lord You have a bigger plan and purpose than I can see. Please save me from ever falling down that pit again. Help me trust you." I have since remembered the impact of that prayer. I still pray it to this day!

Now I had reason to pray that same prayer as we waited for my breast screen results. I was entering unchartered territory and uncertain terrain regarding my own health. I had not been this way before, and I needed to guard my heart if I was to get through this unscathed.

Heart Filters

Amongst the most significant things the Lord has used in my life, are what I call 'Heart Filters.' In Proverbs 4:23 we read, 'Above all else, guard your heart, for it is the wellspring of life.' I distinctly remember my pastor, Lance Lambert, preaching on this verse, the day I was water baptized when I was about fifteen. It made a deep impression on me as he elaborated on its importance, but I didn't appreciate how imperative it would be as I do now!

'Guard your heart.' How do you do this? I suppose there a few ways to interpret this, but for me, it has been by making sure I have fine mesh filters placed around my heart. I have three strong threads out of which they have been woven. These are definitive absolutes that, by the grace of God, I have resolved to guard protectively so they will be firmly in position and operational at all times. They have kept me from falling apart on many occasions. They still do!

These are my concrete convictions:

➤ God is Sovereign. He is Lord and therefore, He is in total control of my life. Because He is God and I am not, I can trust Him 'whatever.'

➤ God is good and everything He does is good. His loving kindness is over all His works and that includes me, in every aspect of my life.

➤ There is nothing that can touch my life, that is not first filtered through God's Father-heart of love for me.

43

I have found these three heart filters to be the most incredible blessings. They have prevented many doubts from penetrating my heart. I wished I'd had them in place when Matt became so ill as a child and my faith was severely shaken. Yet, through the years, they have become absolutely foundational and wonderfully functional.

Now I would have to ensure these filters were well reinforced and daily in use, so unbelief would not seep in and clog around my heart. It wasn't going to be long before I'd know how effectively my heart filters were working!

CHAPTER FOUR

The Moment of Truth

The weekend I spent waiting for my biopsy results went by like 'an asthmatic ant climbing up a hill with heavy shopping.' (A line admittedly taken from the show 'Black Adder' that has become a colloquial expression in our house!) To anyone looking from the outside, I probably appeared to be functioning normally. However, I was more like a duck on a pond, gliding across the surface while paddling frantically below. 'Oh God help, Oh God help!' What if this really is cancer? Breast cancer! That's a death sentence, isn't it?

Paradoxically, even though I felt as if I was swimming for my life, I was also aware of being carried in the current of God's love. I knew the Lord was with me and none of this had taken Him by surprise. He had loved me before He even made the world and had always known His plans and purposes for me. The previous medical tests had implied the news might not be good, but I still sensed the undergirding strength of God's peace. All the same, I was still in a battle. Trusting in God's faithfulness was imperative because my feelings were so precarious.

When the day of the doctor's appointment finally arrived, Len came with me. I was so thankful for his loving support. I wondered how he was feeling. Such a potentially dreadful diagnosis is a major trauma to deal with for any husband. Len is generally a vibrant and willing communicator with anyone, but during the last few days he had been unusually quiet. However, he reassured me "Darling, I will love you and support you no matter what."

"But what do you think about all this? What should I do?" I asked searchingly.

"Let's wait and see what the diagnosis is. Then we'll talk to the Lord and be led by Him. Father knows."

One great characteristic Len has (amongst many), is that he is amazing in a crisis. His rock-like trust in God has been a continual strength throughout our marriage. His ability to make me laugh and see the funny side of things has diffused many awkward situations, for which I am truly grateful.

This day was no different. As we drove in the car, we chatted about everything, without getting too serious about anything. (More great diversional therapy!) Len parked the car and then we took the lift to the top floor of the breast-screening clinic. A knot tightened in my stomach as I remembered my awful day here the week before. My peace was rapidly dissipating while we sat in the waiting room. Well, this was pretty much the reckoning day I had dreaded. Now here I was, like a helpless lamb ready for slaughter!

Eventually, I heard my name called out in a professional, yet monotonous tone. I suppose it was understandable, although some semblance of sympathy would have been great; maybe a kind word or a look of compassion. I guess they'd seen it all before. I was just the next one on their list. We were guided indifferently into a small office to wait and see a doctor we had never met before.

When he arrived, he briskly foraged through my medical notes and then looked up to catch my eye. I read his expression before he spoke and instantly sensed what he was about to tell me. The biopsy and ultrasound scan confirmed that I had ductal carcinoma. It was still in its infancy, but enough to be a threatening problem. There were also indications that the right breast was heading the same way. Calcification was lurking there already. He returned his attention to my file, avoiding the obvious discomfort of the moment.

Just as I was beginning to process this new information, with all the implications of such a confronting diagnosis, the strangest thing happened. In fact, it was quite surreal. The loudest siren I had ever heard began wailing through the building, as if to echo the cry of my own heart. On and on it screamed, filling every chamber in my head. Honestly, what more could go wrong? Now there was a fire alarm and everyone had to bail out of the building. The timing

47

of this was unbelievable. Even a scriptwriter could not have written 'action' at a more inappropriate time. My life had just been put on hold. Now we were running out of the clinic, not knowing whether we were about to be engulfed by flames!

Doctors and patients all made a dash for it together and waited outside on the tarmac, equally bewildered. The physician who had just diagnosed me with cancer stood with us and about fifty other confused people, until we were told it was safe to re-enter. It helped dispel our consternation briefly, that's for sure! However, Len and I were soon back in the same clinical office (as we had been earlier), ready to discuss the prognosis for the rest of my life.

"Where do I go from here?" was the inevitable question to my new doctor. This was unfamiliar territory to me. I didn't know what to say. He looked at us with empty eyes and sounded as somber as an executioner. What should he say at a moment like this? I assume it wasn't easy for him either, but he was the doctor! Surely, he would help steer me in the right direction. His only suggestion though, was to contact the hospital urgently and speak to the breast specialist in the public health system. Evidently, he was not qualified to give any further advice.

Oh, thank you so much! Now I had a million questions rushing through my head all at once. What would the treatment be? Might I need surgery? (O Lord, surely not!) Would I need radiation to stop the cancer spreading further? Should I have chemotherapy? Could I lose my hair? I felt like a pressure cooker at boiling point. I wanted answers to my questions but apparently, he couldn't help alleviate my concerns. The advice for my treatment would all depend on the specialist at the hospital. I would have to make an appointment. "Goodbye!"

It's an interesting observation, that when patients are treated for shock or trauma of any kind, they are usually wrapped in a warm blanket, kindly reassured and closely monitored for any significant changes. How good it would have been if there was such a protocol to treat the emotional shock of being diagnosed with cancer. How I longed for someone to reach out with comfort and understanding. If there wasn't a warm blanket available, just to be cocooned with compassion would have been wonderful. Nevertheless, we sat in an air-conditioned chill that momentarily seeped into my soul.

A few minutes later, I slumped down into the front seat of the car, stunned with disbelief. Seriously! Did a truck just run over me? I couldn't have felt more flattened, even if one had. Initially, Len and I were quiet for a while, allowing the gravity of the situation to sink in. Then, as if in unison, we both suggested that we should pray and commit this whole situation to the Lord. We needed Him now, more than ever.

It seems that it doesn't matter what circumstances you might have faced before, the current one is generally the most pressing. It certainly was this time! I remember saying, "Lord, I don't know if I will live through this, or die. But, whatever the outcome, will you use this to glorify You somehow?"

Len joined with me. "Yes Lord, be glorified in us and through us. Help us to walk through this holding each other's hand, knowing that You hold us both in Yours."

I cannot recall the rest of the journey home. I was too numb! We arrived safely but as we got out of the car that day, I was aware that a new season was just beginning…and this was just day one!

CHAPTER FIVE

Our Dog Mollie Teaches Me a Lesson

Would God *really* allow me to have cancer? Maybe if I prayed and everyone I knew prayed, I would wake up out of this nightmare and my life would return to normal. I knew my Heavenly Father had a perfect plan for me. That had never been in question. But surely, this wasn't it! I prayed it wasn't! Nevertheless, there are times when fathers just know, in the best interests of their children, they may have to decline their fervent requests.

An illustration from our little dog Mollie comes to mind. Right now, she is sitting at my feet. Mollie is the sweetest little thing and she touches my heart every day. That is the problem. She has these big kohl black eyes that widen each time there's the slightest rustle of a packet that could possibly contain food.

At the moment, I'm taking a break, having dinner. Mollie was fed a few hours ago, but seems to have forgotten. Now, she's staring at me intensely, trying to make me feel guilty. You doggy lovers know what I mean. However, she oscillates from cute and cuddly, to being overweight (she's a foxy cross). As she's getting older, her finely structured legs aren't coping with the added calories very well. Consequently, we have to stop giving her the 'little extras' that she loves so much.

This is very difficult! To turn away from her pleading requests and deny what she lives for, is hard. I love her. We all do. Each one of us would gladly give our scraps in response to her tail-wagging antics. We want her to be happy, so the temptation to feed her is there constantly. Yet if we did, she'd continue to expand and as a result, she would limp with pain. Because we love her, we'll want to do what's best. Sadly, that means resisting those longing looks she's famous for, and kindly rationing her meals.

In fact, there was a day I took Mollie to the park and I didn't know she had discovered a secret food source. Because she doesn't have the sense to stop eating when she's full, she ate the scraps that a kind but insensitive neighbor had thrown over their fence for the birds. No one told Mollie she wasn't a bird, so she gobbled the lot, thinking they'd been left there just for her! I was unaware she had already eaten, so I filled up her bowl with the usual amount of food.

Anyone watching her swallow her dinner, would have thought she was starving. As she does, she wolfed it all down in a couple of seconds. Nothing surprising about that. The speed with which she eats has always been phenomenal. Suddenly though, she started to whimper plaintively. As her distress intensified, she began to whine persistently. That caught my attention straight away. "What's wrong with Mollie?"

I felt all over her, looking for an injury. Maybe it was a prickle in her paw? I caressed her stomach. Well, this was some distended abdomen! Seriously, how far can skin stretch? Instantly, I ran down the road to the neighbors I suspected were the culprits; the ones who insisted on feeding the birds in the park each afternoon. What was in the food pile? Were there bones she might have eaten that had punctured her stomach? Is that why she was crying out in such pain? "No," my neighbors assured me; "It was only mince. Nothing that would have hurt her at all."

Ah, now it all made sense. Mollie was so bloated, that she was lying on her side, panting and unable to walk! Thankfully, I realized her condition was not terminal. Her pain would pass, even if it was uncomfortable for a while. Fortunately, no vet would be necessary. She loves her food. But, what she wants and what she needs are two completely separate issues.

How often it is the same with us. We want to be happy. Surely, God wants us to be happy as well. So we plead with Him, promising to do this and that if He answers our requests. After all, God loves us, doesn't He? We forget it's *because* He loves us so much, that He graciously saves us from ourselves when necessary. For this reason,

He may not always instantly answer our prayers in the way we think He should, and give us our heart's desires.

We've put Mollie on a diet now. Unfortunately, that means we must say "No!" You can read her disappointment like headlines on a newspaper! Unfortunately, she doesn't appreciate the love that is behind our seemingly unkind actions. Alas, her eyes look down, she lowers her tail, and skulks away as if we didn't love her. How wrong is she? We can't communicate that to her though, so she's left sad for a few minutes and then all is forgotten…until the next meal!

If only we could realize how much God loves us. It is because He knows what is best for us, that He doesn't always give us what we want, exactly when we want it! Sometimes we may have to wait for a while. At other times, the most loving answer He can give us is "No!" But, when we know how good and kind He is, we will be able to trust Him in the situations He allows us to go through.

This was a lesson I was just about to be reminded of…again!

CHAPTER SIX

Day 2 of the Rest of My Life

So I had just been diagnosed with cancer. What? In my opinion, the actual diagnosis has to be one of the worst parts of having cancer. It's like being catapulted onto a different planet, where the atmosphere is so completely foreign, you need a life-support system just to breathe! Somehow, I slept that night. What a perfect escape from the trauma of the day. Sleep! That blissful state of being totally unaware of what just happened; that peaceful comatose condition which ends all rather too soon, when you first open your eyes and remember it wasn't all a dream. How I wished it was. My reality was only just dawning on me.

For Len and I, the most meaningful part of our day is when we read God's Word and pray together in the morning. I can't begin to recall the countless times the Lord has spoken to us and the Holy Spirit has comforted our hearts as we have rolled our cares on Him. And this day was no exception. We didn't have to think twice before giving this heavy millstone to the Lord in prayer. What a relief to know that He not only hears, but also answers our cries for help.

I have already referred to George Muller in a previous chapter. You may have heard his testimony, how God answered his prayers to feed and clothe thousands of orphans and build homes for them in the 1800s. Muller went through some of the most severe trials.

He wrote, "I have had the most perplexing matters, but I have committed them all to Him. I have sought His guidance, His help, and He has carried me through them all...By prayer and faith, I have had the joy of proving that God does keep His Word." In his times of greatest need, he believed God's promises and depended upon His grace. God never failed him once.

I wanted to have the same testimony of God's goodness and faithfulness. George Muller was just a normal human being, but one who had chosen to totally trust God. He'd experienced miracle after miracle in the most incredible ways. The Bible says that God is the same; yesterday and today and forever. He has always been a God of miracles. Now I needed one. Len prayed with me, as we joined our hearts in prayer, asking the Lord to fulfill His purposes in me, whatever they might be.

At that point, I had no idea how all this would play out. I didn't know what to expect. The intensity or the length of the journey was unpredictable. The doctor I had just seen hadn't given me any game plan or prognosis. The only One who could give the peace I needed now was my Heavenly Father, who I knew loved and cared for me immeasurably.

Hearing from God

I remember reading a book that was of great help to me when I was at the beginning my journey with cancer. *Praying through Cancer* is a 90-day devotional for women, written by Susan Sorensen and Laura Geist. It made a huge impression on me as I turned its pages, soaking up the wisdom of other women, as they battled with their fears and confronted this life-threatening disease.

One thing that had impacted me greatly, was the importance they had placed on specifically hearing from God in their *own* hearts. How it had comforted them greatly. How they had found guidance, direction and wisdom in making decisions about their treatments. It had brought them God's peace in their darkest moments. I knew this was vitally important for me now. Len and I were committing the situation to the Lord daily. However, rolling our burdens on the Lord was one thing. It was entirely different to seek Him, taking the time to listen for His voice and wait for His wisdom. Would God speak to me and give me the direction and assurance I needed? I desperately wanted Him to, yet I've been in many situations where I have prayed about a problem and not heard from Him explicitly. Often I've had to walk by faith, trusting in His written Word alone.

There's a verse in Isaiah that has encouraged me over the years: 'Who among you fears the Lord and obeys the word of his servant? Let him who walks in the dark, who has no light, trust in the name of the Lord and rely on his God' (Isaiah 50:10).

There are seasons when the Lord may not feel as close to me, when He may hide His face so I'll learn to trust Him more. Walking by faith means that we won't always be able to see with our natural eyes, or comprehend with our own understanding. Sometimes, the way ahead is dark. I feared this might be one of those times.

"Oh Lord," I prayed, "please show me what to do. I've never been down this road before. I've no idea what having cancer is like, let alone knowing what to do, now I have it! Will you speak directly to my heart, so that whatever happens to me, or whatever treatment I have to endure, I will walk through this with Your peace."

I was becoming more and more desperate to hear specifically from the Lord. Len and I kept praying I'd make the right decision, and that my heart would be at peace. Yet, God's personal word to me remained so frustratingly elusive!

CHAPTER SEVEN

Decisions

I had no idea that the decisions and choices before me would be so varied and complex. I thought the doctors would make it easy and tell me exactly what treatment I needed. After all, they deal with cancer on a daily basis. Surely, it would be clear to them. I seriously hoped so, because it felt as if I was trying to find my way through a thick heavy fog!

The first thing I needed to do was make an appointment at the hospital. I was told that the earliest the specialist could see me was in four weeks' time. That seemed like forever! Little did I know that during the next few years, on numerous occasions, I would have to wait much longer. "Still," I thought, "Surely they understand this is urgent. After all, I do have cancer!"

One month later, Len and I were sitting with the surgeon, keen to hear his advice. So, I was surprised when he gave me my options. Options? I hadn't planned on options! I'd expected him to explain specifically what he felt was necessary. The familiar knot tightened in my stomach and frustration began building behind my normally calm exterior.

His mechanical manner was hard to comprehend, when every emotion in me was screaming for compassion and understanding. Words of disbelief sprang from my heart and landed in my mouth. Fortunately, something about his appearance cautioned them and thankfully they remained silent!

"Heather, I cannot advise you what you should do," were his first unhelpful words of insight! Maybe the color did drain from my face, but *steel* came into my eyes. The tone of my voice tightened as I articulated my concerns.

"But I've come to ask for your opinion about which treatment is best, because you are now my doctor and I've no idea what to do! What advice would you give your wife if she was in my position?"

"I'm sorry but we can't give our own advice," he repeated with tedious monotony. Now, I know doctors need to be cautious with the recommendations they give, as suing the medical profession has become a full-time occupation for some people! Nevertheless, I was becoming extremely perplexed. It felt like I was hitting a brick wall. "But I can explain your options." Oh, that word again. "Options!" Forget options. I want guidance. Please!

As if he were repeating lines he had rehearsed so many times before, the doctor proceeded to give me my options:

1) I could have radical surgery on one breast, where the cancer had been found, or preferably both, as calcification had also been detected in the other breast. Oh no! A double mastectomy! That sounded horrific to my sensitive imagination. How would I find the inner courage to face that? Eagerly I wanted to explore the other possibilities.

2) They could give me a partial lumpectomy (less radical surgery and more localized surgery). This would reduce the possibility of cancer spreading to other parts of my body. However, with that option, there were less guarantees.

3) Some lymph nodes under my left arm (or perhaps both arms) would be removed, to find out if the cancer had already spread.

4) After the lumpectomy, I could have radiation treatment. This would reduce the prospect of cancer returning. But, once again, no guarantees.

5) Depending on whether my lymph nodes had been affected, I could have chemotherapy, but I wouldn't know that until the nodes had been biopsied and checked. Chemotherapy? Wasn't

that when your hair fell out and you felt so awfully sick? How would I cope with that? Well, I decided right there and then. If I loss my hair, I would buy the most gorgeous wig I could find and treat myself to a new look! Long, wavy, thick blond hair. That might be cool.

6) I could have surgery and radiation if the doctors recommended taking further precautions. Sounded excessive to me! Now my mind was working overtime and my imagination was making this look more like impending torture. There surely had to be another alternative. What was option number 7?

There wasn't a number 7. That was it!

Really? It felt as though the doctor had taken his tennis racket serving for the match and just aced the ball firmly back into my end of the court. The decision was now up to me. Apparently, it wasn't his job to help choose which one or combination was preferable. It was now up to me to go home, do my own research and revisit him when I had come to some sort of conclusion.

Once again, I left another doctor's office, feeling emotionally numb. Actually, numb isn't bad at times like this. You can't feel the frustration and confusion that you might, if you had all your senses alive and functioning normally. Yes, numb is good! Perhaps it is God's way of prescribing anesthetic without painkillers. The trouble with painkillers is that they wear off. So does numb. Eventually you have to come back to reality and face the reason why you initially went into shock. Oh, that's right, I am dealing with cancer. I need to reach a conclusion and no one else can help me. Now I'm dealing with scary. Reality finally dawned on me after about an hour. If only 'numb' could have lasted longer!

Eventually, the 'doer' in me kicked in and so I started planning. I would search out some other opinions. I immediately booked in to see my local GP. She was a compassionate doctor who would hopefully understand my confusion. However, even she hesitated to guide me. She explained how difficult it was, because everyone's decisions were so personal. But as a woman herself, she suggested that surgery would be the best idea. There wasn't as much risk of the cancer reoccurring, so she thought. That was not what I wanted to hear! I was hoping she might have seen the benefit of the less radical treatments. "Oh well," I thought, "this was only her opinion. I knew another doctor. I would ask him."

He was also initially unsure. Seriously, what was the problem with everyone? Why couldn't they be more decisive? Nevertheless, after further consideration, he thought that having radiation would be enough for now. But I didn't want "enough for now!" I wanted the cancer to go away so that I didn't have to deal with this potential killer eating away inside of me. What was it about the 'C' word they didn't seem to understand? Was this doctor hesitant because he felt sorry for me? He had always been so kind and considerate before.

So, now I had one doctor recommending radical surgery and another suggesting the less invasive option. Perhaps I should at least consult with one of the top breast surgeons. Hopefully, they would give me more specific advice. Without delay, I rang their office and expressed my dilemma to the receptionist. "Could I please see one of the specialists as soon as possible, because I have some extremely important decisions to make?"

"Yes, of course, we would be happy to help. But unfortunately, Christmas is just around the corner and we are fully booked up. The earliest appointment would be when the doctors return from their break. Would January 8th be okay?" Her words hit like hailstones. I suppose it would have to be. What choice did I have? I confirmed the date in a disappointed tone and put the phone down.

Another heavy blow! Don't they realize what it's like to have cancer? It was clear I would have to wait again! (Waiting is not my greatest character trait, as you may have gathered!) So, I would have to go through the holidays without coming to any final conclusions. Why were the answers to my questions so hard to find? How could I be happy and celebrate with everyone when I felt as though I was incarcerated on death row? I was beginning to buckle, overwhelmed by an avalanche of apprehension.

I don't remember much about that Christmas. I muddled my way through somehow. It may have looked as if I was functioning normally, but inside I was shrouded by uncertainty. It felt like I was driving a car that was stuck in second gear when I was used to fifth gear. That was normal! We exchanged gifts as usual, but only God could give me the one I longed for most – my health.

We spent a week away with some of our friends. Great therapy. Laughter and activity helped fast-forward the long days until I could see the specialist who would hopefully help me decide on the rest of my future.

Eventually the time came and we arrived in Brisbane, ready to receive the advice I so desperately needed. Finally, I might find the answers to my questions. We were guided into the crowded waiting room. After a while, a nurse called out my name. We followed her to a small room, glad that my suspense would soon be relieved.

When I addressed the doctor who I assumed was the specialist, he preempted my disappointment by informing me that he was only the Registrar. The 'big chief' was still on holiday. Apparently, I was seeing his young intern. Once again, words of indignation queued up behind my teeth. I bit my lip.

Where was the specialist who was going to look at my X-rays, read my reports and give me the benefit of his vast wisdom and expertise? Who was this baby-faced practitioner who looked as if he was just out of school? I silenced my disappointment as I tried to concentrate on his glib comments. After a few brief moments of deliberation, he concluded that either radiation or surgery would be advisable, and that it was really up to me, after all!

The rising indignation I had cleverly concealed, now searched for a terminal of departure! This was my life he was supposed to be considering, not just deciding what he wanted for dinner. If it hadn't been so serious it would have been funny, but this was no joke. I was devastated. I made my way home like a leaf tossed about in a hurricane, unsure of where I might land.

Valuable days had been lost over the Christmas period, while waiting for the doctor in Brisbane to give me his unhelpful advice. By now, the cancer could be freely roaming around inside me. Who knew what kind of damage it might be doing? I needed to go back and talk to my surgeon as soon as possible. Perhaps he could be more definitive now and help me reach a conclusion.

There was one issue though. I still hadn't heard from the Lord and time was running out. I was about to decide whether or not to have the radical surgery and I didn't want to make such a significant decision alone.

I kept asking Len what he thought I should do. But how does a husband answer such a question? He wanted to support whatever decision would ultimately give me the greatest chance of survival. He could make suggestions, but ultimately it was my call. In fact, that was the same predicament for all my friends and family. How was it possible to be loved by so many, and yet feel so alone at the same time?

When the day of my appointment arrived, I asked my surgeon the same question as I had on my previous visit. "If your wife had breast cancer, what advice would you give her? I've done so much research and I'm still not sure." I could see the strain etched on his face. I'm sure he realized that I wasn't leaving this time without an answer. Reluctantly he proffered a response.

"Heather, if you're pressing me, I would recommend you have the bilateral mastectomy. I know it's the more radical approach, but it's the safest in the long term. I've seen many women needing even more extensive surgery because their cancer has returned later. It's probably not exactly what you wanted to hear, but that's my honest opinion."

My heart paused between beats. Well, that was it. My surgeon had just confirmed what I instinctively knew already. Was this really happening? It all seemed so surreal. In the next few moments, I was handed the form to give my consent for the surgery every woman fears. Apprehensively, I signed. There it was. My signature in black and white. Done!

CHAPTER EIGHT

The 'Path of Life' for Me

One thing still concerned me, as we somberly made our way home. I had signed for the surgery without directly hearing from the Lord. I wasn't entirely sure I had made the right decision, although I was resigned to the fact that theoretically, it seemed the best option for me.

I remember recording a quote from the book *Through Gates of Splendor,* written by Elizabeth Elliot. Her husband Jim was one of five missionaries, killed by Indians in Ecuador. In his own journal, he had noted that when he prayed about his future, he sensed going to Ecuador was God's will for him. How did he know? Because he had felt his heart instructing him in the night seasons. He longed to be so saturated with the oil of the Holy Spirit, that he would be ignitable and burn as a flame for God. Jim knew without a shadow of a doubt that God was speaking to him. There weren't visions or voices, just the counsel of God in his heart. That was what I longed for. The different doctors with their varying opinions had only dug anxiety deeper into my soul.

My friend Bernie sent me a letter one day which included a few scripture texts. One specific verse leapt out at me, about waiting on the Lord and being courageous. I felt encouraged to keep waiting for The Lord's direction. After all, He had known me before I was born. Even though I didn't know my future, He did. I wanted the knowledge and assurance of God's will for me.

The morning after signing the consent papers for my surgery, Len and I had our prayer time together. We were reading through the book of Acts and had come to the second chapter. These were the words we read in verses 25-28;

'I saw the Lord always before me.
Because He is at my right hand,
I will not be shaken.
Therefore, my heart is glad, and my tongue rejoices;
my body also will live in hope,
because You will not abandon me to the grave,
nor will You let Your Holy One see decay.
You have made me to know the paths of life;
You will fill me with joy in Your presence.'

What reassuring words they were to me that day: 'My body will live in hope…paths of life…and joy in Your presence.' I had the sense that the Lord was indeed with me but, was it possible to know His *joy* at a time like this? I was about to find out.

Each morning, Len and I also walked our puppies around the park, just across the road from where we live. On this particular day Len was busy for some reason, so I took them on my own. Actually, it was good. It gave me some quiet time to think over my decision. "Lord," I questioned tentatively, "have I made the right decision? I am still feeling unsettled. Please quieten my heart and fill me with Your peace."

Immediately after I had finished my request, the answer came as a bolt from heaven. Distinctly, I heard the words almost audibly, as if someone was standing next to me, "This is my 'path of life' for you" (from the text in Acts 2:28). That was it! I knew unmistakably, that this was the Lord's word to me. (It was similar to the time I felt God speak to me before Len and I were even dating, when I clearly heard the words, "This is the man you are going to marry!" I have to say I didn't need to be told twice. I was a willing accomplice!)

The most amazing thing happened right at that moment. The Lord gave me such a profound knowledge that this was His purpose for me, and His way of saving my life. A deep peace came into my heart and a joy I could almost taste! And with His reassurance came the faith and courage I needed to follow Him on that path. It really is almost impossible to describe what it's like to hear God's voice.

It's just a deep inner knowing in the depths of your spirit, that God has spoken to your heart, and with it comes such peace!

Here I was, walking around the park whilst sampling the most incredible joy and relief, when I should have been feeling so afraid. This was life-changing for me! If I hadn't experienced it, I would not have believed it was possible. Words alone cannot even begin to describe the inner transformation that immediately took place. It was as if a light had shone into my heart from heaven and instantly dispelled my consternation. Joy, like a golden sunrise, dispersed the dark clouds of dread, strengthening me to face the coming ordeal without fear.

This was the miracle I had been waiting for! I almost ran home on air! This was God's path of life for me, and in *that* I could trust. I had left the house with such a heavy burden weighing upon me, but I returned with a new buoyancy of spirit. The women who had written about walking through cancer were so right. Hearing from God makes all the difference.

It certainly did for me that day!

CHAPTER NINE

"D" Day Draws Nearer

One of the most incredible things about the peace that God gives, is that it doesn't evaporate at the end of the day. Now this does not mean that I'm immune to suffering and sorrow. Not at all. God's joy doesn't stop you from being real and experiencing human emotions. Nevertheless, in the midst of everything, it feels as though there is a bubbling fountain deep inside of you; a heavenly spring of hope that overflows in the most unbelievable way.

The reason I am sharing this experience with you is not to say how amazing I am. On the contrary! I think by now you will have gathered that I have had and probably still do have many questions and trials that keep me leaning heavily upon the Lord. I could never have walked this journey without the incredible healing presence of

God in my life. I just want to encourage you in your journey as a fellow traveler, to seek Him and not to be afraid.

Jesus often said to His disciples "Fear not!" Life can be a scary business. Sometimes, much to their dismay, storms appeared from nowhere, even threatening their very lives. On one occasion, Jesus told them to sail to the other side of the lake. They didn't expect to be caught in a hurricane that day. Yet, fierce winds whipped around them and crashing waves terrorized their battered boat. But they didn't drown!

We read in Acts 27, that the apostle Paul also found himself on a ship that was stricken by surging seas and cyclonic winds. On a perilous journey to Rome, bound as a prisoner for Caesar's court, he had warned the crew to dock their vessel and wait for calmer conditions, otherwise there would be trouble ahead; shipwreck, loss of cargo, and danger to their lives! But they didn't listen. Who was Paul anyway, and what would he know? So, when massive breakers threatened to sink their boat, Paul wasn't in the least surprised!

The storm raged relentlessly for fourteen long nights. If only they'd heeded Paul's advice not to sail, they would have been spared the pending disaster. Darkness landed upon the frightened travelers like vultures of dread. Would they live or die? They didn't know. But Paul did. The night before, God had sent an angel to strengthen and encourage him "Don't be afraid, Paul, for you will surely stand trial before Caesar! What's more, God in His goodness has granted safety to everyone sailing with you." Consequently, he gathered the sailors together and told them, "So take courage! For I believe God. It will be just as He said" (NLT). Miraculously and just as God had promised, all of them reached land safely. Not one of them was lost.

An incredible strength saturates you when you hear from God personally. The comfort of His word in any given situation changes everything. Darkness disappears and fear takes flight. Inwardly you are fortified to face whatever it is you must go through outwardly.

God didn't prevent Paul from experiencing what it felt like to be shipwrecked. But, He did save him out of the disaster, and gave him a story to tell of how he made it to the shore alive. I prayed for a similar outcome. My life was being threatened. But my trust was in the Lord, either to save me from the surgery, or give me courage to go through it, whichever was His will.

There was still time though, for God to miraculously heal me, so I wouldn't have to face the surgeon's knife. However, the closer the day came, the more I realized that God was probably not going to deliver me from the 'fire' but walk with me through it, as he did with Shadrach, Meshach and Abednego when they went through their own fiery trial. The curling flames were heated up seven times hotter than usual, ready to burn them alive, all because they refused to bow before a narcissistic king. I related to what they said to him, as they faced their uncertain future;

"If we are thrown into the blazing furnace, the God we serve is able to save us from it, and He will rescue us...*But even if He does not*..." (Daniel 3:18).

Bravely these men walked amongst the flames, yet their faith didn't flicker and they didn't flinch. They were cast *into* the fire and God brought them *out*, unfettered, unbound and unharmed. Not one hair on their head was singed, their robes were not scorched, and there wasn't even the slightest smell of burning on their clothes. What an amazing miracle!

Their secret? King Nebuchadnezzar said it best when he leapt to his feet in astonishment: "Did we not cast three men bound into the midst of the fire? … Look! I see four men loose…and they are not hurt, and…the fourth is like the Son of God" (Daniel 3:24-25 NKJV). God's presence changed everything, strengthening them to face the flames, whilst shielding them from the scorching heat, at the same time. My prayer was that God would do the same for me.

January 29th arrived sooner than I would have liked. This was the day of my pre-operation interview with the anesthetist. Later, I would be required to answer a million questions from a nurse who had never met me before, who was not likely to see me again, and probably had little or no understanding of how I was feeling. Facts and figures were exchanged and written down in my medical file which was becoming thicker than a thesaurus by the minute. I had been told when to arrive at the hospital, which floor to come to and what I should wear. Once again, that familiar numb sensation began to filter through my emotions, helping me cope with my impending reality. Was it now only three days before my operation?

"Lord, please strengthen me now. I need You to help me even come back here. Nevertheless, You said that this was Your 'path of life' for me. I am so thankful for this offer of life. Settle my heart again as I place my hand in Yours. I'm so grateful that You are with me. Help me glorify Your name as I face this coming ordeal."

When the interview was over, I picked up my folder of hospital information, suppressed my anxious feelings and took the lift to the ground floor. It was so good to come out of that sterile atmosphere and into the sunlight for the rest of the day. I drove back home with my thoughts on 'automatic.' I already had way too much to process, and my mind was having difficulty making the leap. Fortunately, there were a few more days of relative normality, and I was going to make the most of them.

I booked myself in for a relaxing massage, went to the movies and enjoyed going out for lunch with one of my girlfriends. Keeping busy was great diversional therapy; useful emotional beta-blockers that helped close the door on the daunting images trying to infiltrate my mind. The unconditional love and support from my family was a constant source of encouragement. It was also reassuring to know that so many of my friends were praying. Gradually, the same peace that came when God spoke His Word to my spirit, swept over me and trickled gently over the riverbed of my heart.

CHAPTER TEN

"D" Day Arrives

And so it was that February 1st arrived, unannounced to the rest of the world, but written in large letters followed by an exclamation mark in my diary. I'd packed my hospital bag the night before, so when the alarm rang, rousing me from my safe cocoon of sleep, I didn't have much to do except shower and coax myself to get into the car.

I wasn't allowed to eat because I was fasting, so breakfast was out of the question. Strangely, I really missed my food that morning. (Somehow the day always seems brighter once I've eaten!) So, to be denied any comfort food on this of all days seemed quite heartless. However, I understood the reasons of course. Len was unusually quiet as he drank his cup of tea. Well, what do you say to your wife, knowing she's about to be carved up and her femininity stolen from her innermost being? He couldn't prevent anything I was going to face that day. I expected that his imagination was working overtime as well as mine. Watching someone you love suffer needs almost as much grace as the one who is suffering. You are hurting together, just in different ways. I was so sorry he had to go through this drama with me, but then, that's all part of the marriage deal; "For better or for worse!" It's what love does.

Len started the car and I slipped in beside him. I had already decided that I would rather he didn't stay with me at the hospital. I had to have the radiation dye flushed through me and hot needles placed in strategic areas to help guide the surgeon's knife. I felt that we would be better left to our own thoughts and prayers. There is nothing worse than sitting in the waiting room making small talk, when you want to think serious thoughts!

I didn't need Len by my side as proof of his love for me. That had always been a given. He would have sat with me willingly, but I preferred him to pray with me and drop me off at the hospital. Then, at least he would be free to occupy himself with the regular duties of his day. He needed diversional therapy too. (I didn't have to ask him twice!)

Len hugged me and gave me a big kiss, reaffirming he would always love me no matter what. No mutilation or humiliation would ever change his love. Now, it doesn't get much better than that for a wife! How grateful I was to have married such an understanding and affirming husband. He knew just the right words to say and the most precious words to pray. Soon it was time for me to get out of the car with my little case and say goodbye. Parting with the most knowing and loving look, he waved and drove off, merging with the rest of the traffic. Quickly, he was gone.

To an onlooker, it might have seemed as if I was standing there alone. But I wasn't! An amazing strength surged through my heart as I opened the door into the X-ray waiting room. I was aware of the Lord's presence in the most profound way. He was walking with me on this 'path of life' and I knew that we were going through this together.

I assumed that I would have to wait (that's not rocket science), so I had packed my journal and a pen to help keep my mind firmly focused on the job at hand. I wasn't one bit interested in looking at pictures of beautiful women on the front pages of the well-worn hospital magazines. I was preoccupied, psyching myself up to be anything less than beautiful for quite some time. I didn't need to be mourning my losses but rather thanking God for this operation that I believed was going to save my life.

I just wanted to quieten my heart and lose myself in my own thoughts, but firstly I had to be prepped for the radiation dye that was to circulate throughout my body. A nurse offered me a hospital gown to change into and then asked me to take a seat and wait to be called. Waiting again! "Get used to it," I thought, "This isn't the first time, and it certainly won't be the last!"

It wasn't long before my name was called. I braced myself as the dye was injected but fortunately, it didn't hurt. I returned to the waiting room and found the same chair I had been sitting in, just a few minutes earlier. Still in my gown and feeling quite ungainly, I prepared to gather my scattered thoughts and write them into some kind of orderly formation. Hopefully, they would make sense one day when I had reason to revisit them. Today, I just wanted to talk to God and feel the sense of His love wrapping around my heart. I consciously made up my mind to block out the world for a while. I would be jolted firmly back into reality soon enough.

I had chosen a special book for this occasion; gold leaf on the outside and textured to hold. I opened it purposefully and stared at the first blank page. How do you start to journal on a day like today? However, my mind was soon busy and my pen seemed eager to fill the empty space. Before long, my thoughts spilled over and covered the first page with ink…

"This is a monumental landmark in my journey through breast cancer. What a bumpy ride it's been! Today is the day of my double mastectomy. I've just had my radiation injections to test the lymph glands before my operation. I'm sitting alone in a tiny waiting room; alone with the Lord and my book that I've been reading the last few days: 'The Five Silent Years of Corrie Ten Boom' by Pamela Rosewell Moore. I am about to gown up for my X-rays and I've just finished the last chapter, which just about sums up how I am feeling. Corrie had often said during the difficult circumstances of her life, "It is not so much what happens, but how we take it that is important." Over the years, she'd noticed

82

an interesting principle, which is so encouraging; "The deepest fellowship with Him lies in not resisting when suffering comes our way, but in going through it resolutely with Him. Don't wrestle…just nestle!"

Psalm 91 is also a wonderful comfort to me. "Lord I'm nestling under the shadow of Your wings! Cover me Father with Your hand. Let me experience all You have required for me to experience and shield me from anything unnecessary. Be my refuge and my shield. Fill me with Your joy, because You have carried my sorrows. You have assured me that this is Your 'path of life' for me, so please hold my hand as we go through this together. Thank-you for Your whispers of love today. I love You Lord. Be my strength and fill me with Your courage to go through this now!

Thank-you, Father."

~~

I was still writing, content in my own private world, when I sensed the presence of someone walking towards me. Somewhat startled, I looked up to see a familiar compassionate face. My friend Mel had come especially to be with me, while I was waiting. How incredibly kind. But then, I knew something about her that many didn't. She had also been diagnosed with breast cancer, the previous year. As we were talking in the doggy park one day, whilst walking our respective puppies, she had mentioned how having cancer had changed her life. Mel's breast cancer had radically rocked her world.

In the light of her experience, I knew that Mel was one person who could understand the apprehension I was feeling. She wanted to shoulder the burden with me in the most loving way she knew how. I have thanked her many times, but I don't think she will ever fully realize how much it meant to me. Someone who had also been diagnosed with breast cancer was here with me.

"Heather, I didn't want you sitting here alone, knowing what you have to face today. I just wanted to come and sit with you. Is that okay?"

Of course, it was. It was such a kind and thoughtful gesture. I had completed what I was writing in my journal, so I closed it with an air of finality and we began to talk together. The minutes passed like seconds. Friends can transform the ordinary into special, and that's what she did. I believe she was sent by God, though she might not see it that way! Does that matter? Not at all. All I know is that it meant the world to me.

I can't remember how long I waited as we were so absorbed in our conversation, but I was quickly brought back to reality when my name was called. It was time to have the X-rays. Mel understood what that meant. She had done her job and knew she couldn't travel with me any further. She gave me a hug and waved goodbye. The nurse then walked me into the next part of my day.

The initial part of the procedure wasn't painful, thankfully. All good so far. Perhaps it wasn't going to be so bad, after all. Wrong! The X-rays were going to show where they needed to place various hot wires into the parts of my anatomy that were going to be taken from me. However, I needn't have worried. Fortunately, these days they don't let you suffer. They kindly injected me with some local anesthetic and proceeded with the job in hand. Sometimes it's best not to overthink technicalities, so I returned to my familiar safety of 'numb.'

The medical team assigned to me for this part of my procedure were especially sympathetic. I smiled and they tried to mirror my optimism, although I felt I was teetering a bit at this point. I hadn't been aware of a procedure quite like this before. I just remember being bandaged like an Egyptian mummy around my upper torso, with the long wires poking out, too lengthy to be concealed by the surgical dressings. Thank God, no one could see me now. What did I look like? Something out of Star Wars maybe?

No one warned me I would have to leave the clinic and make my way across the highway to the hospital looking like this! A nurse came with me, helping to distract my total humiliation. She chatted to me as if this was the most natural thing to do; to cross the street, looking like I was held together by wires. I only had to walk a few steps but it felt like a hundred miles! Thankfully, my embarrassment quickly subsided and I was soon safely hidden behind the doors of the pre-operation clinic.

Now there were formalities to go through. Hospital papers had to be filled in at the counter, saying who I was and why I was there. Seriously, I hoped they knew! I certainly did. I fumbled through one of their magazines, keeping my mind from vivid thoughts that were flying around inside my head. At the same time, I knew the Lord was standing at the gate of my heart, with the sword of His word firmly drawn across it. This was His 'path of life' for me. He was helping me not to be afraid.

I was relieved when they eventually called me. I wanted time to pass quickly, so I was glad to be kept occupied. I was interviewed by a gentle nurse. It's interesting how you notice these particular characteristics in people when you are feeling vulnerable. Kindness, compassion, and understanding are rare qualities, but invaluable in moments like these. She tenderly explained the process that I would be going through, and her eyes leaped out as if to embrace me.

She then sent me off to the changing room, to slip into one of those attractive hospital gowns with the paper hat and slippers, and tight elastic stockings! If only the congregation of our church could see me now. No makeup and no accessories apart from my wedding ring, which they tied up with tape. I caught a glimpse in the mirror and looked incredulously at the sight before me. Lovely! I felt like a lamb going to the slaughter! At least though, I would be unaware of the carving knife!

Now all I had to do was climb into the hospital bed reserved for me, lie there (and hopefully stay there), until it was my turn. I remember this moment so clearly. It is etched precisely as with an artist's chisel, carved deeply into my heart. This had been one of my fears. I had wondered how I was actually going to have the courage to get myself onto the bed and lay myself down without jumping off before they wheeled me into the operating room. Would I really be able to go through with it? I wasn't so sure.

However, the most amazing thing happened. Even though I had rehearsed this scene in my mind many times before, I hadn't expected to feel God's presence in such a tangible way. Words alone cannot describe the peace and joy I felt. This must have been what the apostle Paul meant in Philippians 4:7 when he spoke about the 'peace of God that transcends all understanding.' Here I was, being given a heavenly anesthetic from the divine dispensary. I imagined myself walking along the 'path of life.' I was so grateful.

I thought about my trip to the Philippines a year earlier, when I had visited the destitute people who lived on the rubbish dumps. They didn't have hospitals like this and doctors offering them free surgery. What could the women do there? They probably would not even be able to get a diagnosis, let alone have any hope of living through it. Here I was, so blessed to be receiving the best of care.

I didn't have to wait long before I felt my hospital bed begin to move. They had come to take me away! Two wards men, one at each end of the bed, helped steer me towards the next season of my life. We made our way down the cold, sterile corridors. Two large flap doors opened into a much smaller room. (No going back now!) More kind people were already there to help me on my way. They wrapped me up in a large preheated blanket which felt so good. The wonderful warmth seeped into my body and wrapped around my heart. More importantly though, I was engulfed in God's love.

The anesthetist gently took my hand in his. Then came those words that cause you to hold your breath momentarily, "This might sting a bit!" Generally, this is a huge understatement, but it wasn't so bad. "Heather, count back from ten for us, will you?" Well, I had never excelled in the math department, but I figured I could help them out in their calculations. "10…9…8…7…" and that was all I remember, thankfully!

CHAPTER ELEVEN

Recovery

Thank God for anesthetics! My mind does not need to know, neither does it want to know what took place on the sterile slab that day. Len and I had prayed that my surgeon would remove every cancer cell. He was also going to take out some lymph nodes from under my left arm to see whether the cancer could have spread to other parts of my body. In prayer, we filtered everything through the fact that my life was in God's hands and we knew that was the safest place I could be.

The operation lasted over three hours. Then, from somewhere close by, I vaguely began to hear a muffled voice. "Heather, you're awake now." I am so glad someone told me, because I wasn't too sure at that point. I certainly did not equate how I was feeling with being awake or hardly even being alive. Yet apparently, I was. I must have drifted in and out of consciousness for a while. However, the seriousness of what had just happened soon dawned upon me. Back to reality once again! But, no pain as yet. So far so good. Thank God for drugs in times like these. The nurses kindly reassured me that I would be kept as comfortable as possible and they were as good as their word.

It wasn't long before I was wheeled to another ward where I would spend the next few days. But, as the hours slipped by, I could not understand why I was still feeling so ill. Surely, this drugged up feeling should have worn off by now. I had an intravenous drip in the back of my hand and I had been told that if the pain started to bite, I should press the buzzer. It would automatically inject some serious painkillers. That sounded like heaven to me.

After a couple of days though, I still felt unwell. Why wasn't I bouncing back as quickly as expected? Walking to the bathroom became a massive effort. I felt faint and wheezy. Where was the old Heather? No one told me this was part of the deal. Surely, it would pass and I'd be better soon. But I wasn't.

It was sometime during the second day after my surgery, that I felt myself slipping into some sort of vague unconsciousness. My strength was draining from me, as if my life force was being sucked out of my bones. I was in trouble. I reached for the bell to alert the nurse on duty. All I could do was to whimper weakly, "I think I'm going to faint!" Then came the call that everyone dreads, whether they are the patient or not: "Code blue, code blue!" which basically lets everyone in the hospital know that someone is in need of some serious help.

Suddenly, I was surrounded. Nurses and doctors came from everywhere. Pandemonium! They rushed the emergency trolley to my bedside. A kind nurse positioned herself at my head, stroking my forehead, while whispering in my ear, "Heather, it's going to be okay. Hang in there!" I didn't seem to be hanging on to anything. When you're slipping away from life, there is nothing much you can hold on to. The word 'slipping' implies that whatever is happening to you is completely out of your control. There was nothing I could do. Everything was being done for me.

A doctor began pumping the carotid artery in my neck. Was he trying to kill me? I thought that I was doing a pretty good job of dying anyway, but it felt as if they were helping the process along very nicely. Then they beat upon my chest. *Careful!* I'm wounded there, can't you see? Could this really be happening to me?

While all this was going on around me, I started to feel myself drifting away. Strangely, I remember thinking how close this was to the anniversary of my dad's death, the year before. Perhaps I might be seeing him again soon. Heaven here I come! Voices around me became muffled and I remember seeing what looked like a softly lit entrance of a tunnel. I was being drawn towards it, but I only had a momentary glance, because whatever the doctors were busy doing prevented any further travel along that pathway.

My heart was beating so fast. Faster than ever before. (When I asked the nurses later, they said that it had been pulsing at 220 beats per minute!) Now I must say, I am not an exercise enthusiast, so my heart is not used to racing that fast. Between 60-80 beats per minute is usual for me, so this was bizarre! It wasn't out of rhythm, as in atrial fibrillation, but it was pounding so rapidly, I thought it was literally about to burst. They injected me with some medication to try and quieten my heart, but nothing had any effect. My heart just would not stop its manic pace. It kept beating like a metronome on speed!

I can't recall much of what happened next. Our memories are clever when it comes to blocking out trauma. All I know is that I woke up in the heart ward on the ninth floor of the hospital. When I looked around, I noticed that I was the only one in the room and I had my own individual nurse. That was not a good sign!

My heart was still aching and thumping in my chest. The thick cannula needle in the back of my hand stung. How I wished I could rip it out, but I needed it for the liquid drugs they were giving me. For the next eighteen hours my heart hammered inside my chest, with a will all of its own. It was unstoppable and unforgettable!

My immediate family were the only visitors allowed to see me at this time. I knew they would be worried but they kindly concealed their concern. They didn't stay with me long. I couldn't muster the strength to speak and they couldn't find many words to say, except how much they loved me and that they would be praying for me.

(How grateful I was to have a family who would pray, when I felt too weak to say much at all – to them or God!)

I was so sore! Pain pulsated from my surgical wounds. In fact, heaven began to seem quite an attractive option. Would I ever fully recover? It's scary feeling so vulnerable. I hadn't been prepared for this! But then, without any prior indication, the throbbing suddenly ceased and blood stopped rushing through my head. Relief washed over me like a torrential downpour. My strength surged back, along with a sense of well-being again.

Now let me encourage any of you who are reading this, and may be facing any kind of major surgery. My experience should not be considered 'normal.' I had overlooked to let the anesthetist know that occasionally I have heart palpitations. I hadn't had any recent occurrences, so I didn't think to mention it. I had no idea it would be such important information. I won't forget again. The key is to tell the doctors everything you know about any condition you have, even if you think it's irrelevant.

It may well save you going to heaven prematurely!

CHAPTER TWELVE

Back to Some Kind of Normality

One of the greatest rewards after this dramatic saga was the freedom to have a shower. I'd been attached to all kinds of drips, which had made showering prohibitive. How I had longed to feel the warm refreshing stream of water, washing away my fatigue and despair. It seemed as if I had been in hospital for an eternity, when in actual fact, it had only been three days! How do you use up so much adrenalin in such a short space of time? No wonder I felt completely exhausted.

Eventually though, I was wheeled out of the coronary care unit and taken back to the surgical ward. A room had been prepared just outside the nurse's station. Fresh sheets, new scenery and soft rays of sunlight were waiting there to welcome me. My daughter Hannah was a nurse at the hospital and knew some of the staff on the sixth floor. They had found out that I was Hannah's mum, so I sensed they were giving me special treatment and caring for me with extra kindness.

It wasn't long before the most beautiful bouquets of flowers were arriving with my name attached. More came than there were vases available, so we squashed the bunches in together. You could have been forgiven for thinking that I had been dropped off at the perfume section in a classy department store. It was as if someone had come with expensive bottles of fragrance and sprayed them all around my room! I imbibed the rich aromas before they wafted out of my room and into the rest of the corridor.

My wonderful friends had been praying for me, and word had traveled about my complications after surgery. Sending flowers was their way of hugging me when it was too soon for them to visit. It was going be a while before the tenderness would subside, allowing anyone to get near enough, even for soft hugs. Nevertheless, I was content to be sitting up in bed in this sunlit room. Finally, I could see that the light at the end of the tunnel wasn't an oncoming train! Perhaps I would be able to go home soon.

I picked up my note book that had been left unopened for the last few days. While I was preparing to write, a little key fell off my bedside table. Its tinkling sound caught my attention. What was this key doing on my cabinet? It wasn't mine. Where had it come from, and to whom did it belong? (I never did find out.) But suddenly the thought occurred to me: There are keys to coping with cancer! It was a timely reminder. God has given us keys as we go through our different trials, enabling us to unlock unlimited amounts of joy and faith. I asked the Lord to show me these keys during my next season of healing and restoration. I gathered my thoughts and then picked up my pen.

"Today is day four since my operation. How relevant was the verse in the book of Acts that the Lord handpicked for me just prior to my surgery; 'My body will rest secure' was the same verse the Lord impressed upon me when the code blue alert went off and the emergency team rushed around my bed. The Lord held my heart in His hands and shielded me from the fear of the trauma.

Thank-You, Lord for answering my prayers during these last twenty-four hours, when I called out in such desperation. My heart is beating back in its normal rhythm and my temperature has come down. Thank-you for being my deliverer when I've felt so weak and in so much pain. Thank-you for the gift of this single room and all these beautiful flowers; Your creative masterpieces that color my world. Thank-you so much. I am so very grateful."

~~

I was even more grateful when the day came for the drains to be removed from under my arms. Finally, I was free to go home. Two days earlier, I could never have imagined leaving so soon. But it was bittersweet. I was coming back to my family, yet my son was still very ill and I knew he would need my help. How was I going to cope? Would I be able to manage? (It's hard as a mum because even though you know you shouldn't be picking up washing, vacuuming, and wiping down bench tops, you still feel the need to do it anyway.) Could I sit on my hands and resist helping with all the household chores? Well, I'd soon find out!

My friend Mandy came to the hospital to visit me, only to find that I was being discharged. She got there just in time before I left. So, instead of sitting on my bed chatting, she gathered the flowers, helped pack my bag, sat me in a wheelchair and steered me towards the hospital entrance. She is a typical 'doer'! If anything needs fixing or sorting, Mandy will organize it with absolute grace and ease, and even make it feel like fun (even though it's not). Len was there with me too. He tried to do whatever he could, but every time he turned around to pack something, Mandy had done it already. She had got there first!

Len drove me home and Mandy followed in her car. She must have overtaken us though, because when we arrived, she'd already made herself at home in our kitchen and was making the proverbial good old English 'cuppa' tea.

Caring friends from our church and neighborhood sprang into action straight away. During the next few days, meals were dropped off at our door, wrapped country-style in tea towels and arranged attractively on wooden trays. What a smorgasbord of delicacies we enjoyed, baked with loving care and a myriad of spices. My heart was full of gratitude to the Lord, for surrounding me with such love.

I didn't have any pain yet, thanks to the drugs. However, it wasn't long before the uncomfortable sensations began to bite and more medications were needed. This was to be expected after the surgery I'd just endured, so I felt quite unashamed to have as much help as was necessary, to keep me pain-free for as long as possible.

The ability to sit on my hands for any length of time didn't last long. I must admit that when my family wasn't looking, the urge to bend down and pick up washing or straighten the bedclothes was way beyond my good intentions. I refused to let them see me wince, my determination wouldn't allow it. They still don't know, so please don't tell them!

I was well and truly bandaged with some sort of sticky plaster around my chest, therefore I had no idea what the damage would look like. I dreaded facing the mirror. Would I look like a mutilated mess? The extent of it I couldn't begin to envisage, nor did I have the emotional fortitude just yet. That could wait a few more days. I was happy with that!

CHAPTER THIRTEEN

Facing Reality

I was so thankful to be home. There is nothing quite like it. Even when you have travelled all around the world, most people say they are very glad to be back in their own beds! (Now I know I am comparing home comfort with hospital beds. It's like contrasting a bed in the Versace to one in a motel! There's really no comparison.) But add to that the home cooking from our friends and the warmth and laughter of our crazy family, not forgetting our puppies Mishka and Mollie, and the picture is pretty well complete.

There was still something bothering me, though. Surreptitious thoughts crossed the canvas of my mind, painting potentially awful possibilities. I tried to visualize what I would look like once all the bandages had been removed. It was hard to imagine, so I attempted to block out the imagery. Nevertheless, the day had to come sooner than later. And so it did! What would Len's reaction be? This was going to be a huge leap for him, as well as me. Amputation is serious business! I had no idea how I would feel. I tried to prepare myself psychologically for the imminent 'moment of truth' and asked God to strengthen me. I especially needed His help today.

I purposely chose to go to the hospital alone. I wasn't sure of how I would feel, and so preferred to deal with my unpredictable emotions privately. I was expecting a fountain of tears to flow from my well-hidden fears. Len totally understood and would have done anything to help, but really, what could he do? What could he say?

I was able to drive the car myself by this time. At least, I would get these hot sticky bandages off my skin. I arrived at the clinic for my appointment. Waiting this time was no easier than at any other time, when the outcome is still unknown. "Lord," I prayed, "please be with me." I knew He was. He promised He would never leave us. Thank God for that. I needed His peace and courage to fill my heart once again and help me face this part of my journey.

My name was called, and tentatively I followed an elderly and matronly nurse. Whether she had been run off her feet that day or was just way past her use-by date, I don't know. Maybe some nurses just become jaded and fed up with seeing so much sadness. Anyway, she just ripped off my bandages as if she was in a hurry to catch the next train. Secretly I thought, "Wow, go careful love. Do you have any idea what you're doing?" I was seriously doubtful.

As I stood before her, feeling bruised, sore and self-conscious, she curtly told me I could get dressed and go home. And that was it! I stifled my protests into silence until the shame of the experience had dropped below the crest of my indignation, and thankfully left without embarrassing myself. Fortunately, there wasn't a mirror in the room. Even if there had been, I knew I was not ready to process the facts, so it didn't matter. Right then, I couldn't have even cared. I would deal with that later.

How do people develop such wooden feelings? A friend once showed me a fossilized piece of wood that had literally turned to stone. Had this nurse's emotions become fossilized over the years? Maybe! Seeing so much trauma, pain and sorrow can possibly make us impervious, for our own emotional protection. Suffering softens some people, but can harden others. Soft would have been great. Someone with kid gloves, not steel gauntlets!

As soon as I left the clinic, I took the lift to the ground floor, landing like a wounded bird with an injured wing. I made my way home, although my feathers were still ruffled. I was smarting badly on the inside and extremely tender on the outside, but immediately Len's gentle embrace helped to flush out my frustrations. I snuggled into my nightdress, purposely avoiding the mirror, and jumped into bed. It would be a few more days before I could look at the scars the surgeon's knife had left behind, let alone show them to Len.

After a couple of days, I summoned the courage to assess the damage. I knew that the Lord had been with me, strengthening my heart, and this moment was not going to be any different. Cloaked with His love and comforted by His presence, I felt ready to face my reality. Surprisingly, as I surveyed my landscape, what I thought would be unsightly rugged terrain was not nearly as horrific as I had imagined. The surgeon's careful carvings would eventually heal and the impact on my spirit was unbelievably negligible.

I am so grateful for the fact that my self-esteem is not bound up in my physical appearance. My sexuality does not come from the size and formation of certain body parts. I know that I am so loved by God and this makes all the difference. It's not something that is just theoretical knowledge. It really is a love I experience daily.

I hadn't always felt this way. Growing up during my teenage years, I'd felt very insecure in who I was. I didn't feel beautiful. I'd grown up in a Christian home knowing that I was dearly loved, but positive comments about how I looked or presented myself were frugal. My parents had grown up in those post-Victorian years when it was doubtful that the word affirmation' had even found its way into the English dictionary. Understandably, my mum and dad were products of their own upbringing, and I was a product of theirs.

Humility was a prized virtue in their opinion that needed to be encouraged as much as possible. However, Ma and Pa had no idea how much I longed for a compliment after having a haircut or when I occasionally wore a new outfit. Money was tight in those days and so when I was in my mid-teens, my mother made quite a few of my 'Sunday dresses.' As I recall, my school uniform felt at least three sizes too big, but that was so I could grow into it! The hems of my dresses were a few inches below my knees, whereas my friends wore theirs inches above their knees. I felt like a missionary in training!

I think that's why I wasn't in any hurry to learn to sew. I didn't appreciate Ma's labors of love and the long hours she spent making our garments. I should have been a lot more thankful, but I wasn't. I couldn't wait to earn my first meagre income so I could buy my own clothes. Trousers, for the females in our family, were frowned upon, however I set about changing that point of view. Jeans were in vogue. Everyone else had them, so I made sure there was a pair hanging in my wardrobe!

During my high school years, I wore the brand of shoes called Hush Puppies. If you are English, I am sure you will feel profound compassion and sympathy. No heels for me! They were suede shoes bought for comfort, but certainly not for fashion! My long straight hair was parted down the center of my head like a runway for British Airways, in contrast to many of my friends whose hair was cut more stylishly. I couldn't help feeling so different. Longingly, I admired the good-looking girls, comparing myself to them unfavorably.

Trendy clothes were not a top priority in our house. It was the inner beauty of a quiet and gentle spirit, we were reminded, that was important. The only trouble was, I was neither particularly quiet nor gentle! I think if I had asked my parents what I was like growing up, they would likely have said that I was highly spirited and enjoyed a challenging debate at their expense, (which could be interpreted as being argumentative!) That being fairly accurate, my upbringing was probably more like the masterful 'breaking in' of a young filly. (The use of a bit and bridle was going to be far more effective than just a juicy carrot!)

Now I realize that I am writing this from my perspective and not theirs. Because they loved me so much, they wanted to protect me from an overinflated opinion of myself. I am thankful for this now and genuinely appreciate their concern. Nevertheless, I still felt very average throughout my teenage years. I couldn't ever imagine being married. Wasn't it the beautiful people who were chosen for marriage? All on my own I worked it out. I would be a missionary. So, I placed a large map of India on my bedroom door at college to remind me of future possibilities. Maybe God might want me, even if no one else did at the time. (Albeit, there were a few later!)

Therefore, when I met Len, he blew me away. He actually told me he thought I was beautiful! Many times he repeatedly expressed his delight in me, but my reply would bounce back "No I'm not!" One day, he reacted to my predictable response, "Maybe you don't realize, but it hurts me when you don't receive my compliments. I love you so much and you are very beautiful to me. Can't you accept that this is how I feel about you?" Suddenly it hit me! I wasn't used to so much attention and I thought I was being humble to react like this. Of course, I loved every minute of it. What woman wouldn't?

Len's continual expressions of love and encouragement to me have been like water falling onto parched sand. He didn't just say,

"I love you darling" when we first met. He has made it his quest to remind me daily and I have never tired of hearing those words! They always melt my heart and clothe me again with the feeling of being special to him. I am so blessed to have a husband who understands how fragile a woman's sense of beauty is. We are like fine porcelain china, but if our feminine self-esteem gets bumped, our emotions can shatter into slivers and shards. Beauty is something we admire in each other. We long to feel attractive. We value soft skin, flowing hair that frames our faces and makeup that helps us look great, even if we don't feel it!

Then there are times when we look and feel less than lovely. Instead, we flat line through the day. Our hair hangs limp, clinging mercilessly to our heads. Our kohl eyeliner runs unkindly down our clammy cheeks. Consequently, we don't feel as good on such days, and it affects us.

On the other hand, when we are dressing up for a wedding, or doing our makeup to go out for dinner with friends, we love the way it makes us feel. All glamorous and gorgeous. What a difference it makes. Kind compliments from special people in our lives stroke our sense of value, and inside we glow. Appreciation fertilizes the seeds of love inside our spirit, that grow in the soil of life.

I am so grateful for God's love, and the affirmation He has given me through Len. As a result, I was not as deeply impacted by my double mastectomy as some have been after their breast surgery. I've been heartbroken to hear of women who have been abandoned by their husbands at such times. Instead of being supported, some are left to face their journey alone. Love is meant to be a comforting light that shines in the darkness. How extremely sad when that light is extinguished. How bleak is the darkness then!

In 1 Corinthians 13 we read:

'...If I have a faith that can move mountains, but have not love, I am nothing...Love is patient, love is kind. It does not envy, it does not boast, it is not proud. It is not rude, it is not self-seeking, it is not easily angered, it keeps no record of wrongs. Love does not delight in evil but rejoices with the truth. It always protects, always trusts, always hopes, always perseveres. *Love never fails.*'

What a perfect description of love! When a woman is diagnosed with breast cancer, this is the kind of love she needs; understanding reassuring, affirming, comforting, accepting, caring and enduring. Just for her loved ones to be with her, offering an encouraging hand that expresses, "I'll walk with you on this journey whatever it takes, no matter what you go through. I'll love you regardless of what you look like and however you feel."

This was the gift of love that Len gave to me at the time when I felt the least lovely. He didn't make me feel ashamed or disfigured. On the contrary! He was so gentle and never demeaning in any way. Therefore, I was able to accept the reality of what had happened to me in my own time. Love is the best environment in which to heal, and understanding is the most favorable atmosphere in which to flourish. I was grateful for both.

It also helped me greatly to know that I was scheduled to have reconstructive surgery down the track, so I wouldn't always look like this. Hope is a marvellous narcotic. I took it in generous doses and it certainly helped to sedate my sense of self-consciousness. Everything had been set in place to 'rebuild the ancient ruins' and so for now, I just had to mend. However, that was going to take time.

I didn't realize how much time!

CHAPTER FOURTEEN

Prognosis

There were still unanswered questions at the forefront of my mind, that clamored for attention. I didn't know if my lymph nodes had been infected with cancer. If so, had it spread further, how far might it have ventured and what other damage could it have done? These were huge considerations I attempted to delete when slipping into sleep. What was the purpose of lying awake worrying? I would deal with the facts when I had them. Until then, I'd try not to superimpose my fears onto the private screen of my imagination. (Sometimes it worked!)

Eventually, the time came to revisit my surgeon. I remember the growing feeling of uncertainty as I sat outside his room. I had brought along a good book to help relieve the predictable boredom of waiting again. My appointment was scheduled for 5:00pm. The specialist had been operating all day, so his secretary warned me he might be delayed in getting to the clinic on time. Concentrating on reading though, was difficult. My mind kept wanting to stray down the 'what-if?' paths. I knew however, that this would be like inviting a thousand snakes into my bed, expecting not to get bitten! I didn't want to be infected by such toxic thoughts, so I deliberately avoided the question.

I turned my attention to an older woman sitting close by. Our eyes met and instantly we connected. We understood why we were there; to finally receive our lymph node test results. It felt as if we were waiting for an impending storm to pass, not sure whether dark clouds were going to break over us, or rays of sunlight might sneak out from behind them, and shine upon us. Either was a possibility.

I can't remember if I was called in to see the surgeon before my newfound friend. But I do know that I walked in bracing myself, ready for the following prognosis that would answer the question hanging precariously over my life. I searched carefully to see if my doctor's demeanor would give away any clues before divulging the secret contained in my file. It was hard to tell. I imagine that he had cleverly learned to mask his feelings having spoken to many women in such situations. Kindly, he didn't hold me in suspense. "Heather, your lymph nodes are clear. That is good news!" When the impact of these words had registered, relief unclenched my trepidation. I could breathe again. (I almost hugged him, but he really wasn't that type!) It meant I wouldn't need chemotherapy or radiation for now. He did mention though, almost as an aside, that he wanted me to come back in a couple of weeks for more carving. My biopsy results had indicated that further clearance was advisable.

No problem. I was just so happy to hear my lymph nodes were clear of cancer, that any suggestion of further surgery was fine with me. "Just sign here, Heather and we'll book you in again." I signed without the slightest hesitation this time, and left with more joy than I could contain. I could not thank the Lord enough for His kindness and love to me. I had been given the sweetest reprieve and it tasted so good. Len shared my gift with me. It was our gift. We were going through this together, and our hearts felt the strengthening grace of God in that monumental moment.

As it had been a late appointment, we didn't stop for the usual coffee we might have, had it been earlier. Instead, we headed home. The necessary preparations for dinner had to be taken care of. But at least for now, I was out of imminent danger. I felt as if I had just been released from death row!

The next day I woke up with mixed emotions; grateful for my positive prognosis, but disappointed about needing further surgery. Still, it was important my surgeon felt he had removed everything necessary to give me a clean bill of health. Evidently, he wasn't sure at this point, so back I had to go.

Fortunately, this was not going to be anything like the length or severity of the last operation, except it had only been one month

113

since my 'code blue' experience. I was certainly not keen for a repeat performance, so there were some issues to raise with the anesthetist when I saw him prior to the surgery. Sympathetically, he listened to my concerns and graciously allayed each one.

"Now that we know why your heart reacted last time, we will change the concoction of the drugs we give you, ensuring this will definitely not happen again!" Oh bliss, oh joy! I was so glad to hear this. My heart could relax again, confident the doctors were aware of my condition and I could expect calmer waters for a smoother ride this time.

Two weeks later, I was all gowned up and ready to go. This time, everything went without a hitch and I was discharged within a few days. Now all that remained was to arrange the appointments required for my reconstruction. I looked forward with anticipation to these visits. The specialist was working hard to lessen the visible damage, which helped so much in my recovery process How good it was to look and feel more like myself again.

Everything was progressing well. Each day I felt stronger and life was returning to some sense of normality, although 'normal' is not a word we often use in our family. What is normal? Maybe you have had good reasons to ask the same question!

I had one more appointment to see my surgeon before the new implants would be inserted. But, I heard a throwaway comment in the clinic that caught my attention. The breast surgeon was leaving the public hospital and returning to his private practice. I would not be seeing him again. It was evident he was eager to leave. "Politics," he inferred, as if I understood. Now what would happen to me? It wasn't up to him to choose my next doctor. He couldn't give me any answers, but then, he wouldn't have divulged anything, even if he did know.

The hospital didn't have any solutions either. I was one of the last four patients left helpless in the same situation. Our doctor had done an excellent job amputating our body parts and everything had been put in place to complete our reconstruction, but no one was available to finish the job! We were left dangling in mid-air, on the thin thread of hope that someone would solve our dilemma. None of us had any idea we would have to wait so long!

One of my neighbors was indignant. She was ready to call the TV channels and jump up and down with disgust about the way our predicament was being mishandled. Her anger inspired me to write a calm but assertive letter to the hospital. Could they please provide some help in this unusual case? They responded quickly, promising to outsource a plastic surgeon who would be willing to complete the necessary surgery, and the public hospital would foot the bill.

Now we were reassured. We thought it would be soon, but we could not have been more mistaken. One year later, a letter arrived, advising me to contact a doctor on the Gold Coast who had agreed to put us out of our misery. I could not afford thousands of dollars needed for private surgery, yet this kind plastic surgeon had offered his expertise. I didn't hesitate for a moment. Picking up the phone

115

I snagged an appointment immediately. No way was I going to let this fish slip through my net!

Unfortunately, I would still have to wait a further six months. Non-paying patients are understandably not listed as high priority, but I was just grateful to have been given a date. The involvement of pastoring our church, and caring for our son Matt, who was still ill at this time, meant the months flew by. It seemed as if one minute I was being told that I'd have to wait half a year, and the next minute I was gowned up again. I reminded the anesthetist of my previous dramas, then soon I was counting down 10…9…8…and quickly I was out to it. (I love that feeling of floating away into oblivion, even though you ultimately have to come back to reality!)

I felt across my chest with searching fingers. What would my new appearance look like? After a few days, a nurse removed my bandages, revealing the end product. Not amazing but satisfactory. Nevertheless, I was just thankful for any hillocks appearing on the desert plain. It was good to finally leave the hospital and hopefully stay away…for a while!

CHAPTER FIFTEEN

Round 2

My life resumed with the same intensity, just minus the cancer dramas. I settled back into the well-worn paths of attending Matt's doctor's appointments as we tried to solve the mystery of his complex illness. I was glad to put the past behind me.

However, when twenty months later, I found a small pea-like nodule in the side of where my left breast had been, I was absolutely mortified. Understandably! I'd had a double mastectomy. Hopefully it was simply a cyst and might just disappear. Yet the insidious lump did not recede as I had expected, so I asked my doctor. Thankfully, he thought it was nothing to be concerned about. I felt some degree of assurance, but a nagging concern was still gnawing away at the back of my mind. Why wasn't it going away? What was it?

I confided in one of my friends, who had been a nurse and was following my story closely. "You mustn't leave this any longer," she chided. "Get an appointment immediately to see your surgeon. Remember, it's your body, not theirs. You must get this investigated as soon as possible." She made her point!

I knew that she was right, so I dragged my heels back to the hospital. Not again! Not more tests and humiliating examinations. The specialist prodded and poked, trying to conceal his surprise, but thought an ultrasound might be a good idea. "I'm sure there's nothing to worry about, but let's check it out anyway."

Lying on the X-ray bed, I watched uneasily as the pictures were projected onto the screen. The technician carefully examined the images. Anticipating my concern, he turned to me reassuringly, "I really shouldn't be saying anything until this has been reported on, but if you're asking me (which I was), I am 99% sure that this is just a harmless cyst and nothing that will cause any further problems."

Great! That was exactly what I wanted to hear. My doctor was sure, the specialist was sure, and so was the technician. Confidently, I went back to my surgeon on the second floor who was waiting to review the report. "Seems all good to me, Heather. So what do you reckon? Are you happy to leave it, or do you want me to remove it anyway?" Quick as a flash, I heard the words tumble off my tongue as if the answer had already been conceived within me, "If you don't mind, I think with my history, it's probably best taken out, just to be safe." I was getting used to anesthetics. One more wouldn't hurt.

So another operation date was scribbled in my diary. 'Gowned up and ready to go' was becoming almost as common as getting in the car and going to the local shops!

On the day of my surgery, I knew I'd be placed first on the list. As an insulin-dependent diabetic, fasting through the night could cause my blood sugars to plummet during the operation, so they would need to have me there early. This suited me perfectly. I didn't want to wait around starving half the day.

I knew the procedure well by now. Papers were signed, forms were filled in and interviews completed by the nursing staff. I wasn't worried. Neither was anyone else. It was just a cyst, right? Wrong! This was no ordinary lump. It turned out to be one of the rarest types of cancer! The medical technician testing the biopsy had only ever seen three of these types of cancers in all his years, and he was nearing the end of his career!

What a shock it was to be told that I had cancer for the second time. Who expects to get breast cancer after a double mastectomy? Well, occasionally it happens. Cancer once beaten, can return. The late former British Prime Minister, Margaret Thatcher, said it well: "You may have to fight a battle more than once to win it." It looked likely that's how it was going to be with me.

In her book, *There's No Place Like Hope,* Victoria Girard tells of a time she was once given a card that pictured a teddy bear sitting on the floor with some of its cotton hanging out. Inside the card it read, "Ever feel as if you've had the stuffin' knocked out of you?"

119

I knew exactly what she meant. That day, the stuffing was knocked out of me, for sure!

The word 'cancer' never ceases to pack a powerful punch. The shock sent shivers through my soul. My emotions froze and formed into an ice-block of silence. Stunned, I left the clinic, allowing my feelings to defrost from my fright. I was not free from cancer yet. Now they wanted to take out more lymph nodes to see if this cancer had spread. Reluctantly, I presented myself at the reception desk to book in for my next operation.

As I stood waiting, I could feel warm salty liquid brimming up behind my eyes and sliding slowly down my cheeks. The Bible says the Lord collects our tears in a bottle and records each one in His book (see Psalm 56:80 NLT). Well, He would have been busy on this day. Maybe I had cleverly covered my unspoken premonition that this was also cancer and tears were the release of these private fears. Some things go deep down into our souls and don't surface until they are given permission. Now, I gave myself consent to cry.

I phoned my daughter Hannah, who was in China at the time. She was teaching English to doctors and students in Beijing Medical University. I wanted her to know and feel the comfort of her voice. "Oh no, mum. Not again. I am so sorry! I'll get the church here to pray for you. I love you." I really missed her, but was grateful she didn't have to watch me go through all of this, and at the same time, deal with the trauma our son Matt was experiencing. Fortunately, she was far away.

I didn't tell Len until I returned home. I wanted to share my shock with him personally and feel the comfort of his arms around me once again. There's healing in hugs, like soothing oil on broken skin. I didn't want to bear this alone. Together we would pray and commit the continuation of this journey to our Heavenly Father. This hadn't taken God by surprise. He'd seen this coming. It's just that we hadn't. Nor had anyone else for that matter!

So, back I went to hospital. I needed to have two-thirds of the lymph nodes removed from under my left arm for further testing! Then there was the potential problem of developing lymphedema (a possible side-effect from this type of operation, causing swelling in the arms due to fluid retention). I had heard about this before, as a friend of ours experienced this condition before cancer tragically took her life. I certainly had never anticipated this.

My surgery would be followed by strict rehabilitation. I would have to keep my left arm elevated above my shoulders for several weeks. The drainage of my arm was imperative for a good prognosis and gravity was going to be helpful in the process.

I surrounded myself with a plethora of pillows, propping up my arm whether I was in lying in bed or sitting in the lounge. How uncomfortable and awkward was this! Even walking around in the house, I had to raise my arm. Well, I might as well lift my arms up to the Lord and not waste the opportunity. We are encouraged to lift our hands to Him, so I was already halfway there. I wanted to praise Him no matter what, even though I still had no idea whether

121

the cancer had spread or not. This second cancer had been so close to my armpit, that there was no guarantee there would be clearance this time.

Prayer is such an incredible gift; the privilege to talk with the Creator of heaven and earth. It's a heavy burden to bear when you don't know whether you're going to live or die. Yet the peace that came when we cast our cares upon the Lord was amazing. I would never have thought it possible unless I had experienced it myself. Surely, you're not meant to have this much joy at a time like this. I was experiencing the grace of God in the most extraordinary way. His love was shielding me, so I wasn't afraid.

One Sunday at church, I read a few verses from Psalm 116;

'I love the Lord, for he has heard my voice;

He heard my cry for mercy.

Because He turned His ear to me,

I will call on Him as long as I live...

The Lord is gracious and righteous;

Our God is full of compassion...

When I was in great need, He saved me.'

It is so true! He does help us when we cry out to Him. It's not that He necessarily prevents us from walking *through* our trials, but He strengthens us and comforts us *in* them. I'm not brave at all, but His grace is sufficient. Truly it is!

If my surgeon had the benefit of foresight, he might not have extracted as many lymph nodes as he did. He didn't know that the report on my surgery would come back as normal. Nevertheless, in my opinion, it was well worth going through the procedure to have the 'all clear' again. Maybe my heart did miss a beat while waiting for the words to fall from his lips. But when he gave me the good news, my heart happily returned to its regular rhythm.

Still no chemotherapy required. I could keep my hair. I must say how much I admire those of you who have gone through this. As I have previously mentioned, I had already decided that if I was ever to have chemotherapy, I was going to buy the best wig in town. I imagined the new hair styles I could wear. However, I have also heard how uncomfortable they can be, and you probably don't even care how you look when you feel so awful. I still considered the possibilities if ever the need arose, but thankfully it wasn't going to be necessary.

Once again, I'd been given a most wonderful gift...a reprieve!

CHAPTER SIXTEEN

Radiation and a Funeral

The word 'radiation' didn't register with me straight away, but it soon became clear that my surgeon hadn't finished with me yet. He handed me a referral to contact some of the radiology units. These were private centers however, and there was no way we could afford the $2,000 this treatment would cost.

The alternative though was going to be almost as impossible. I would have to catch the bus from the Gold Coast which took the public patients to Brisbane for their radiation treatments early in the morning and stay there all day until the bus returned. The procedure only took twenty minutes but getting there and back, five days each week would be a nightmare! I was still caring for Matt at the same time, and he needed me on call 24/7. How was I going to be able to leave him during the days, for five consecutive weeks? Hannah was still overseas and Len was busy pastoring the church.

Len and I did what we usually do when we need a miracle; we told God about it. Not that He needed notifying or reminding. He was completely aware of our predicament. He just loves it when we ask Him. My dad often used to say to me, "Heather, Father knows!" meaning that my Heavenly Father had it all sorted, even if I couldn't see the answer. I certainly had no idea, but God did! Amazingly, the solution came completely left of field. Quite unexpectedly, one of our kind neighbors collaborated with a mutual friend. The result of their phone call was the arrival of a get-well card containing a check to pay for my private radiation treatments at one of the best local cancer clinics.

Len and I were overwhelmed. Neither of us knew how God would provide for the miracle we needed. We were praying and yet were still amazed at His provision. We know God loves us. We trust His faithfulness. Then why are we so surprised at the extraordinary ways in which He answers us?

My caring friend had also organized a roster for those wanting to help drive me to and from the hospital each day. I suppose that's what comes with the experience of being a nurse. She understood how sore I would feel and how tired I would become. I was thankful for her anticipation of my needs. She just wanted to be with me on this leg of my journey. Wonderful friends! Here was another angel without wings, although she never saw herself as one! Angels don't have to be huge with golden halos. They are God's messengers, and He lovingly sends them to help us at the most difficult times in our lives. (She didn't know it, or realize the impact of her kindness, but I was so grateful.) Angels incognito!

It had been over three years since my initial diagnosis of breast cancer. Because of the radical extent of my previous surgery, the doctors had not considered radiation therapy as being necessary. It was only after my second cancer that it was recommended. Was it just a sensible precaution or was it absolutely imperative? I asked the oncology specialist. She reassured me in no uncertain terms that this was indeed the best course of action and pressed me to make a final decision. It made sense, so we booked the appointments six weeks in advance for all the sessions I required.

The crisis of cancer never comes at an opportune time. Ever! Ask anyone who has had it. It always comes as a rude interruption. This could not have come at a worse time for me. Our little family was beginning to struggle. Len was now having heart problems and had made a couple of emergency visits to the hospital himself. My dear mum was nearing her end and declining rapidly in the nursing home where she lived. I was visiting her regularly and often. Matt was still suffering periods of unconsciousness and struggling with constant seizures.

We also continued to pastor our understanding and supportive church. They looked on helplessly, longing to be able to help. They did what they could practically and they prayed. Sometimes a tasty meal would arrive on the doorstep. More angel deliveries! My diary was already full with appointments for church and family, let alone trying to fit in my own treatments.

Christmas came and went. We had a fair idea that this would probably be Ma's last one with us. She was deteriorating noticeably; eating like a sparrow and tiring quickly. It was heartbreaking to see her like this. Over the years she had been with me during my saddest moments, tenderly encouraging me and faithfully praying. Now the flame of her candle was about to be extinguished. She wasn't afraid. In fact, I hadn't seen anyone more excited to leave for her heavenly home. Ma used to light up like a Christmas tree when she talked about being with the Lord, and her eyes sparkled with anticipation at the thought of seeing Pa again. She had lived with an ache in her soul since his death that nothing could anesthetize, even though she was grateful that he no longer had to suffer from the frailties of his stroke.

However, I hadn't anticipated that she would leave us right in the middle of my radiation treatments. I was devastated! Her day of departure was a Sunday. My sisters and I sat closely beside her. She was unconscious during the last few hours, nevertheless we wanted her to sense our presence and feel the reassurance of our love. We watched over her through misty eyes and whispered in her ear what an enduring treasure she had been to us. These were our remaining precious moments together, our final opportunity to express how much her unshakable faith and unconditional love had meant to us all individually. We would never forget!

Suddenly though, I had a phone call alerting me to the fact that Matt was about to have a seizure and required my help. It was time to tear myself away. Nothing could have been more agonizing at that moment. The invisible cord between us was about to sever. Tearfully I hugged her, and kissed her goodbye.

I was being tugged by another emotional cord. I was needed at home. My heart could not have been heavier, even if it had been chained to concrete. I waited pensively for the inevitable phone call. It was only a couple of hours until my sister Ruth rang. "Ma's with Jesus! She's gone. She's with the Lord!" She punctuated her words with joyful elation and I shared her relief. During the last few weeks, we'd watched as exhaustion had washed over our mum, No longer could she muster the ability to bounce back. The burning embers in her soul were fading, but her spirit remained as strong as ever! What a wonderful example she had been to our family. "Lord, help me trust You like Ma did. Please keep my spirit strong in You."

The radiation was really starting to bite me now. My skin was erupting in raw welts. I had been told to anticipate this, and warned it would probably get even worse towards the end of the sessions. Gratefully, I lathered copious amounts of creams and ointments on my parched skin which sucked in the moisture insatiably, helping to cool the burning from the blisters.

I had more treatment booked in on the day of Ma's funeral. Kindly, the receptionist gave me an understanding reply, "Oh, I'm so sorry!" and rescheduled my appointment. Radiation and a funeral in one day was seriously more than I could manage!

Len had previously taken my dad's funeral. It had been such an amazing celebration of his life but then he was a remarkable man. The building was packed to the rafters with people who had come to say farewell and express their love. Our congregation knew him fondly as 'Pa.' He was my father, but they all thought of him as their fatherly friend. Ma had been so touched by the sense of joy at his send-off, that she asked us to have the same kind of funeral for her. Same design of coffin, same flower arrangement, same songs, same venue, in fact, same everything!

It was clear though, we could never do a repeat performance of Pa's funeral for Ma. (Fortunately, she wasn't there to know!) Len was unwell, and in and out of hospital himself at that time. I was in the middle of radiation and feeling utterly exhausted. We just unable to do the same for Ma. Instead, our family gathered together around her coffin in a side room at the funeral parlor and shared our most cherished memories of God's gift to us through her life.

Should we have expected a trouble-free funeral? Could we fit in one more drama with everything else going on in our lives? We were about to find out!

After the conclusion of our little gathering, the family were to walk behind the hearse to the graveside where Ma would be laid to rest. However, we were informed that because Queensland was in the throes of torrential rain, Ma's grave plot had become saturated. If it were to be excavated, the heavily sodden soil would fall in. So, Ma was reinstated to her prior position in the mortuary until further notice! Why was I not surprised? (Although I had never heard of this before!) I'm glad she never knew. Thankfully, she wasn't there. She was safely home in heaven, never to feel pain or suffer again. How wonderful is our heavenly hope!

It was three days before one of my sisters received a call from the Funeral Director. "We can bury your mum today but you'll have to hurry. More rain is on its way!" There wasn't time to ring around for the normal graveside service. Ruth rushed in to grab some softly scented yellow roses, then Libby and I joined her and drove to the funeral parlor. Ma could be buried at last. But there was no time to be lost, not even half an hour. Charcoal skies were threatening and thunderheads were building quickly.

The lady official walked with us behind the hearse to the soggy spot where Ma was to be lowered. She positioned a CD player close by and pressed the 'play' button. As the casket descended, the music we'd chosen for this special moment wafted across the hillside. The poignant song *Turn your eyes upon Jesus,* brought heaven to our hearts. We three sisters wrapped our arms around each other and stood melded as one. This was our mum. We had all been influenced by her gentle authority and enduring love. Now we were pressing the 'pause' button. She was gone, but we knew we would see her again.

131

The simple engraving on Ma and Pa's shared headstone seems to say it all: 'Together, forever with the Lord.' Thankfully, 'pause' is not forever. It doesn't mean 'delete.' Now we are on 'fast forward' until our heavenly reunion. Who knows for how long?

CHAPTER SEVENTEEN

The Pause Button

The 'pause' button has also been pressed on my journey with cancer and for that I am so grateful. I've kept my scheduled visits to the breast specialist and I'm doing all I can to stay well. Will I remain cancer-free? Only God knows the answer to that question.

Vickie Girard, in her book *There's No Place Like Hope,* shares her feelings about re-diagnosis. I love her attitude. She says that she has chosen to live her life without trying to foresee all the problems that might loom ahead. It's like going on a picnic on a cloudy day. I agree. Why worry too much about the weather forecast? It may or may not rain. If it rains, you might get wet but until then, make the most of the sun. Enjoy the experience of joyful living. Prepare your food, throw all the gear into the car and go! However, if it does rain, pack up as fast as you can. If you get wet, have a shower when you get home, dry your hair, relax in some fresh clothes and relish the fact that you have some precious memories of a great day. Nothing lost and everything gained.

I remember it was the same with us as kids. Pa would bundle us into his Singer Gazelle (a very old make of English car probably not even seen on the roads today). We would throw in a blanket, an inflatable dinghy, a few buckets and spades and off we'd go to the beach. The fact that it was overcast made no difference whatsoever. We didn't own a TV to check the weather forecast to see if it would be sunny on the south coast of England. We just went.

If it was raining when we got there, we would just shelter in the shops, with a soft Cornish ice cream and a chocolate flake on top. Then as soon as Pa thought the sun was about to emerge from behind the clouds, we would run and stake our claim to a spot on the sand. If it was sunny and warm, we would make the most of every minute. If it was sunny and windy (which it usually was), then we'd just sit on the beach shivering in our wind jackets, determined to enjoy ourselves anyway. And if it wasn't sunny, we'd still have fun. We made sure of it.

This seems to me a great way of dealing with life when you are in remission. Let's keep committing our way to the Lord. It's one thing to trust in the Lord's power when He works miracles for us. It's another thing to bow before His wisdom when we have to walk through dark valleys and don't always see supernatural intervention.

As David writes, in the most well-known psalm of all, Psalm 23 (my comments in brackets):

'The Lord is my Shepherd, I shall not want.' (Even when I was diagnosed with cancer!)

'He makes me lie down…' (on the hospital bed, when I really wondered how I ever would have the courage!)

'He leads me…' (when I had no idea what decisions to make or what I should do.)

'He restores my soul.' (When naturally I am afraid, He heals my heart.)

'He guides me in the paths of righteousness…' (i.e. right paths, especially when the doctors were reticent to advise me.)

'Even though I walk through the valley…of death, I will fear no evil, for You are with me.' ('Even though' are such all-embracing words. They don't fight against the sovereignty of God. They allow us to bend with the winds that blow against the palm branches of our lives.)

'Your rod and staff comfort me.' (When others don't have any idea what to say or what advice they should give, God knows how to lead and gently guide us.)

'You prepare a table before me…' (God's Word has been food for my soul and nurture for my spirit. I have fed upon His love and faithfulness at the most sumptuous of banquets.)

'You anoint my head with oil and my cup overflows.' (I love Eugene Peterson's paraphrase of this in *The Message*: 'You revive my drooping head; my cup brims with blessing.' It's been unbelievable the joy I have experienced through the anointing of His presence.)

'Surely goodness and love will follow me all the days of my life.' (How amazing is this! Everything God does for us is good, and it's always done out of His unfailing love.)

'And I will dwell in the house of the Lord forever.' (Here on earth, I'm part of His family. In eternity, I'm going to live with Him forever. In John 14:2 Jesus reassures his disciples; "I am going to prepare a place for you...And I will come back and take you to be with Me that you also may be where I am.")

In this well-loved Shepherd psalm, the phrase 'valley of the shadow of death' seems particularly pertinent for those who have been diagnosed with cancer. You may be in the fight of your life. Your prognosis might still be in question. If you have committed your life into God's hands, you won't need to fear any evil, for the Lord Himself walks with you. That makes all the difference.

~~

I have shared just a brief part of my story. I hope it encourages you on your journey. I trust that the Lord will comfort you and help you to be courageous in all your struggles. I pray that whatever you are going through, you will never doubt God's love. 'Weeping may endure for a night, but joy comes in the morning' (Psalm 30:5 KJV). In seeing our lives from our own point of view, we may well weep! But I have found that the joy we experience 'in the morning' comes when we also see our lives from God's perspective.

In the next few pages, we will ask some valid questions about the purpose of pain, and search out some life-changing answers. We will always have the best view from God's vantage point. He is the One who created us and He knows the plans He has for us. It has helped me greatly to understand that there is a divine heart of love behind each tear I cry and every trial I go through.

May God strengthen you with His power. May you have great endurance and patience. And may the Lord bless you…abundantly!

Section B
Life from God's Perspective
(An understanding of suffering)

CHAPTER EIGHTEEN

Valid Questions

Sewing has never been my favorite hobby. From my school days when I dropped the pins all over the floor and realized that my seams were never going to come even close to looking professional, I avoided the sewing machine as if it were my enemy.

Hand sewing was different. Somehow, I could mend and stitch with a needle without feeling as if I was going to war. So when we moved to pastor a church in New South Wales, and I met a woman who specialized in making handmade quilts, I asked if I could join her. She made it look like fun. I gathered my materials and psyched myself up, ready for my new recreation. I imagined the beds in our house covered with cottage-like quilts and thought how good they would look. I love country style anything! Day by day I stitched and sewed. Week by week my patchwork production was growing and gradually taking shape.

However, the underside was a real mess; a scrambled mixture of unfinished seams and untidy sections. Knots were clearly visible and threads hung loosely. Nevertheless, from the top, I thought it looked amazing; segments all finished, loose threads hidden and the pattern quite spectacular (even if I say it myself). It took months of work to finish, but I was so thrilled with the result. It covered our bed beautifully. I won't say blood, sweat and tears went into it, yet I felt as though a good part of me did.

We are like God's quilt. In Ephesians 2:10 we are called 'God's workmanship,' a divine project that He is purposefully designing, a unique masterpiece that He is colorfully creating. Philippians 1:6 (NKJV) says, 'He who has begun a good work in you will complete it until the day of Jesus Christ.' Once we have given our lives to the Lord, that 'good work' begins.

We generally see life from our own point of view, yet with eyes of faith, we can catch a glimpse of what God is doing from His perspective. It's wonderful. It broadens our limited understanding. It fills us with hope and helps us trust, when we know whose loving hands are skillfully working on us. Even so, there are valid questions that remain. Sometimes, unsightly threads still hang loosely.

Does God allow sickness and pain, or is suffering entirely from the devil? Is there a redemptive purpose in affliction, or we being punished? Can God's children be under a curse? These are genuine considerations. Many people are confronted by complex situations that leave them confused and perplexed. Sometimes the seams of life come undone and our edges fray. Sometimes life is just messy!

Recently, a well-meaning pastor suggested to Len that our son Matt was under a curse because he hadn't been healed of his illness. (That comment, among others, provoked me to write the appendix about curses at the end of the book!)

Just yesterday, a friend rang asking us to pray for her. She was needing further medical tests because radical changes had shown up in some of her white blood cells. Today, another friend phoned us with the devastating news that his marriage was over. Tragedies and accidents happen. Life-changing losses occur.

As you can appreciate, we often deal with these difficult issues. We are safe if we find our answers in God's Word and His truth is the plumb-line in our lives. If we are genuine Christians, who have put our faith in God, Jesus has absolute power and authority over our lives. His death on the cross was the complete payment for our salvation. Accepting this extraordinary gift of eternal life means that we now belong to Him forever. We didn't earn it or deserve it. It's God's grace-gift. Now we can never be lost (or 'perish'), and no one can snatch us out of His hand (see John 10:28).

Maybe you are reading this and wondering if all of this includes you. Fair question. It is not enough to assume we are Christians. It is absolutely essential to know that we are. A Christian is someone who has been born into God's family by faith in Jesus Christ. That's why the Bible uses the term 'Born Again.' We're born once naturally into the world through our parents; we all have that in common! Then, when God's Spirit drops faith into our hearts to believe that Jesus is His Son, that He died for us and rose again to give us new life, we are 'born' into His family. He breathes His Spirit into our hearts and we become alive spiritually, so we can experience God's love and peace in the most profound way.

Even now, you can pause and ask Jesus to become real to you. Maybe God is filling you with faith at this moment to believe in His Son, and that He sacrificed His life for you personally when He died on the cross. Jesus has taken your punishment! So, immediately you ask Him to forgive your sins, He removes them forever. This is the best news! Jesus has bridged the gulf that once separated you from God. Now you can walk right into His arms without fear. He will never reject you. He longs for you to know His love.

Once we belong to God, our eyes are opened to a new spiritual dimension that we didn't even realize existed. We also discover that we have an enemy who hates what God has done for us! We have been snatched from Satan's clutches. We previously belonged to his kingdom. He didn't bother us then. But, he despises us now, so as a result, he does everything in his power to make us as miserable as possible. He can't rob us of God's gift of eternal life, neither can he separate us from God's love. What he can do though, is attempt to steal our joy and quench our faith. The predominant weapons in his artillery are accusations and lies. Jesus called him 'the father of lies!'

Satan is also described in 1 Peter 5:8 as a roaring lion, looking for those he can devour! Shamelessly, he breathes out wicked and false insinuations about God, casting aspersions on His goodness and how much He loves us. However, we are told to resist him and stand firm in the faith (v9), so we will not be decimated by his deceptions.

I trust that as we look for answers to some of these questions, the torchlight of God's love will shine directly into our hearts and dispel any doubts lurking in the shadows of our lives.

His perfect love casts out fear and His truth sets us free!

CHAPTER NINETEEN

Does God Allow Sickness & Suffering in the
Lives of His Children?

I have shared the tip of the iceberg in my journey called life. I am so aware that you may be going through deeper sorrows than I will ever experience. During many years of pastoral ministry, I have seen some horrific traumas and desperate situations. Every trial we face is formidable. Just in different ways.

My battle with cancer has been extremely challenging. But so has the experience of caring for my son who has an undiagnosed illness that has ravaged his life for over twelve years. Some of these pages have been written while Matt has been unconscious when the only thing I could do was to wait until he took a huge gasping breath as he regained consciousness. Some of his seizures have been quite extraordinary in that they have lasted more than three hours! Then there have been times, he has literally felt he was dying. No doctor, specialist, surgeon, or any other medical physician (and we've seen so many in the last few years that I've lost count), has given us any diagnosis that has led to a cure for his rare condition. Most of them told us they'd never seen anything like this before! (Not the greatest encouragement when desperately searching for solutions!)

I have often said that I would be prepared to have ten double mastectomies if only Matt could be well. But wouldn't any mother feel this way? The worst pain of all has been to watch Matt suffering so intensely, when there was absolutely nothing I could do about it. His story deserves a whole book all on its own. I have no words left to explain the sadness and sorrow I have carried for him. (The Lord alone knows!)

I have also rushed to be with my husband at the hospital after his stroke in 2001, when a doctor informed me that Len was in such critical condition, it was uncertain whether he would live or die. The Lord miraculously brought him through that life-threatening crisis. It would be nearly two years though, before his life would return to any sense of normality. (Only stroke victims and their families know all that this involves!)

Words alone cannot express my deep gratitude to our church for the care and understanding they surrounded us with at that time, supporting us as a family when many others would have chosen to find another pastor. However, when we took into consideration the effects of Len's stroke, and the fact that I have insulin-dependent diabetes, it became quite clear that Len and I could no longer pastor our dearly loved congregation as effectively as we desired. When we prayed about this, we felt the time was right for younger pastors to take our place. Nevertheless, I was heart-broken. It was like having the most precious jewel in my hands and then being asked to give it away. Theoretically I understood the reasons why it was necessary to let it go. I knew it wasn't mine anyway because it belonged to the Lord, but it was still so hard to relinquish what I loved so much.

I share this, not because I desire sympathy. In fact, these trials have been the laboratory where my theology of suffering has been formulated. Over the flames of life's Bunsen burner, my sorrow has been mixed with God's Word. Faith has been tested severely. Trust has been tried under fire. Many questions have swirled around in the test-tube of my heart. Why would God permit our family to go through such trials? Does our distress touch God's heart? Didn't Jesus come to deliver us from evil and give us life more abundantly? Then, was it sin in my life or lack of faith that was the cause of our troubles? However, as the spiritual fires have been applied, I have begun to understand the purpose of suffering from a completely different perspective.

My desire is to share some of these treasures with you in the second section of this book. We will look at some of the lives from characters in the Bible and learn a few of their secrets. We can draw great strength from others who have endured under pressure.

Possibly you may be going through some dark valley. Perhaps you once had faith in God, but everything that has happened to you has gradually eroded away that precious gift. Maybe any flickering embers of hope have been extinguished in the ashes of your despair. Now you wonder if God has even noticed your pain, let alone cares about it. I trust you will be encouraged as you read further, and that He will draw you into His loving embrace.

The story of Noah's ark is a graphic illustration of the security we have when we find our refuge in the Lord. During the torrential deluge, when the Flood destroyed the earth, safety was found by all who entered the ark and destruction for all who didn't. When the rains stopped and the floating home had found a place to rest, Noah opened the window and released a raven. He was keen to find out if the waters had receded far enough so they could disembark. It had been a long confinement. 371 days long! Interestingly, the raven never returned. Open window, open world! Rotting carrion was all this scavenger needed to survive. No need for food back at Noah's place now. So, with unfurled wings and newfound freedom, it took off and flew away.

Seven days later, Noah sent out a dove to check out the flood conditions. Now doves are different. Unlike ravens, they don't feed and float on rank flesh. The dove searched diligently. The mountain peaks had just become visible but the trees remained submerged. There wasn't one branch to be seen. With no food to eat, no place to perch, nowhere to nest and no chance to rest, it flew back home.

One smart bird! As soon as it fluttered by, Noah, who was watching intently, stretched out his hand drawing the little bird to himself and the shelter of the ark once again.

After seven more long days, the dove was sent out on another expedition. Same reason, but different outcome. It still came back, but this time it clutched the promise of hope firmly in its beak; a freshly plucked leaf from an olive tree. The waters were retreating at last! Soon they could leave their restricted enclosure. Soon they could start their new life on dry ground.

One more week went by and then the dove was set free again to find itself a new home. This time it did! A brand-new beginning for this tiny creature meant freedom for everyone else in the ark. They had all been protected from the terrors of the flood, but now they could leave the past behind. God had not forgotten them! They were never far from His gaze and always in His heart. God finally opened the door and out they all spilled. Fresh air! (How good that must have felt!) Fresh start! (How good that must have been!) They could rebuild their lives at last.

There are such times in our lives when, like the dove, we need to return to God's open arms, allowing Him to draw us close until our trials have abated. Then peace (symbolized by the dove carrying the olive leaf) will fill our hearts once again. Never stop searching for answers. Never lose hope. But don't flap aimlessly over troubled waters. Fly back into the safety of God's sovereignty.

Pastor Ray Andrews once said to me, "Heather, in my many years of experience in pastoring and counseling all over the world, I've had to develop three things: a theology for suffering, a theology for weakness and a theology for failure. I could never do what I do today without these three absolutes in my belief system."

When people do not have a theology of suffering they have to blame someone and many times that someone is God! They reason, "It's His fault! He has the power; so why doesn't He use it to heal me as He has in healing others? If God loves me, why am I suffering so greatly?" Sadly, this leaves them wide open for the enemy of their souls to suggest that God doesn't love them, or that He loves other people more. This often triggers a spiritual landslide bigger than any avalanche. Down they tumble, until they are inevitably buried under an icy mountain of bitterness, losing their greatest lifeline – God! Without miraculous intervention, there they will stay, frozen out of the warm embrace of His love. Spiritual hypoxia then subtly creeps in, ultimately suffocating any remnants of faith, and trust in God's faithfulness expires.

Then there are some who conclude that if God is not to blame because He is perfect and cannot do evil, there must obviously be other reasons why they are suffering. "Ah! It's my fault. Maybe God is punishing me for sin in my life, or perhaps I don't have enough faith like others who have been healed. If I come back to God when my faith is stronger, or if I believe harder and do more good works, I might possibly qualify for one of His miracles!"

Is God really like this? Does He use suffering as a punitive measure in the lives of His children? Discipline and chastening? *Yes!* As our Heavenly Father, He is training and instructing us for our good! Punishment? *No!* The judgment for our sins was dealt with by Jesus death on the cross. God punished His Son instead of us. We read in Isaiah 53:5, 'We thought His troubles were a punishment from God for His own sins! But He was wounded and crushed for our sins. He was beaten that we might have peace' (NLT).

In the light of this, let's look at the subject of suffering a little closer. Let's bring up the magnifying glass and examine the story of Job in greater detail. It helps so much when we can see things from God's perspective!

CHAPTER TWENTY

Job's Story

The story of Job is one of the oldest accounts given to us in the Bible and perhaps one of the most fascinating when it comes to looking at life from God's perspective. It is one man's story of unimaginable suffering. Job had no idea why such traumatic events happened to him. However, we are given unprecedented VIP seats in the heavenly arena and as we watch the drama unfold we discover some incredible insights into the purpose of pain. Do good people suffer? Yes, apparently they do.

In Job 1:1 we read, 'In the land of Uz there lived a man whose name was Job. This man was blameless and upright; he feared God and shunned evil.' He was a great man. According to some people, he should have been the last one to go through trials of the kind we shall consider. Job loved God and he did everything to maintain his integrity, love his family and live uprightly in his community. Surely then, God would bless him with a stress-free life to show how He rewards those who are devoted to Him. It would be an easy conclusion to reach unless we had been given inside information to the contrary.

The Bible tells us that Job was the greatest man among all the people of the East. I imagine that means he was both great as a man of God and great as a man of this world. He had faith and fortune. A perfect combination it would seem.

Job is elevated to such a level that we are left speechless just considering his résumé! He'd been blessed with an amazing family; which included seven sons and three beautiful daughters. (A quiver full in anyone's estimation; certainly more than I could manage!) He was also extremely wealthy. He owned 7,000 sheep (plenty of food for feasts and sacrifices), 3,000 camels (for milk and transport), 500 yoke of oxen (to help plow and harvest his many acres of land), and 500 donkeys! Needless to say, he didn't manage all this by himself. Many servants helped take care of his considerable estate.

His children were also well established and appeared to enjoy carefree lives. They often partied at each other's home, feasting and drinking together. Food was plentiful and so was fun. We are told that their father prayed for them regularly. (What a blessing to have parents who pray for you. I know, because mine did. Each day when they were alive, they prayerfully brought us before God's throne of grace.) There could hardly have been a more favored family on the face of the earth at this time. They had everything they needed, and more if required!

So, we are introduced to Job. We like him. He is someone we would like to emulate. However, in just a few chapters, we are given a glimpse behind the scenes, at a drama happening simultaneously in heaven. He didn't know, but his life was about to change forever!

A Rare Glimpse into Heaven

God was having a conference with His angels. As members of the heavenly council, they came to present themselves before Him. However, someone else came too. Shamelessly, Satan filed in with them! He didn't belong in that august assembly anymore, although he used to!

The Bible tells us he once was the guardian cherub, the 'model of perfection, full of wisdom and perfect in beauty' (Ezekiel 28:12). But he became jealous of God's glory. So much so, that he mounted a rebellion and attempted a coup d'état. He thought he could gather a group of like-minded angels and try to dethrone God! His name 'Lucifer' means 'morning star'. He thought he could exalt his own throne above the stars and be like God Himself! Of course, it didn't work. God threw him out of heaven and down he fell to earth with all the other rebellious angels (see Isaiah 14:12-14; Revelation 12:9). So, how he just walked into God's presence that day is beyond human comprehension and seems unbelievably audacious. Did he think he could merge in inconspicuously? Did he suppose that God wouldn't mind him eavesdropping on the heavenly board meeting? God is unruffled by the fact that he's there, but doesn't let it go by unnoticed. Instantly, He confronts him.

"Where have you come from?" Now this is not a question that God asks because He doesn't know the answer. God is omniscient. He knows everything at any one time. But He wants Satan to own up to his antics, and so He shines the spotlight on him. Arrogantly, God's adversary doesn't even address Him personally. Candidly he quips, "I have been going back and forth across the earth, watching everything that's going on."

This is where Satan lives and works now. Earth is his office! He might be invisible, but he's still very busy planning misery and mischief. He knows he will never be invited back to live in heaven. His days of privilege are over forever. He knows he is destined to burn in eternal fire with all the other fallen angels. He is angry. Very angry indeed! Consequently, he's out for revenge! Venomously he looks for ways to poison as many people as possible with his spite and malevolence, making their lives hell on earth! Maliciously, Satan plans their misfortune and schemes their demise.

Many people do not believe in a personal devil, but 1 John 5:19 says, 'The whole world is under the control of the evil one.' We are also told in 2 Corinthians 4:4 (NLT) that 'Satan, the god of this evil world, has blinded the minds of those who don't believe, so they are unable to see the glorious light of the Good News that is shining on them.' He has powers! His name means 'adversary or accuser.' That is where his power resides; in his accusations and lies! (Any opportunity Satan can find, he will accuse somebody, somewhere, of something!)

On this occasion, we find him in heaven's conference room. God initiates the conversation. He's not the One on the back foot when it comes to dealing with the devil. God has a question to ask, and someone He intends to talk about.

"Have you considered my servant Job?" Before Satan can utter even one accusation, God expresses absolute delight in His friend. "There is no one on earth like him; he is blameless and upright, a man who fears God and shuns evil." What a great compliment from the Lord Himself! (Here is one man will hear those enviable words, "Well done, good and faithful servant!")

I have been amazed as I've pondered this scene in my mind. God is the One who highlights Job's wonderful godly character for Satan to consider. Now that's a scary thought! Poor Job. He's doing his best to live life to his greatest potential. When he's examined, he scores the highest marks and is sent to the top of the class! He's a perfect 'A' student. Surely, God will now describe the way in which He intends to bless him. Apparently not! Instead, Job is given the greatest recommendation to the devil himself! Satan barely blinks and hardly draws breath. His answer is already burning on the tip of his tongue.

"Job? Yes, I know Job! He loves You because You love him. You care for him. You bless him. You look after his family. Is it any wonder he loves You? Look how prosperous he is! But, if You take Your hedge of protection away from him and strike everything he has, he will surely curse You to Your face."

In the most unexpected reply, God actually buys into Satan's deal. There is no argument. In fact, it's quite the opposite. God says "All right. Do what you want with all that he has. But whatever you do, *do not* hurt him." In other words, he had permission to take what he had, but not touch him physically. Will Job curse God, or won't he? This is now the million-dollar question. What a scene. What a scenario. What a rare insight into the heavenly realm.

Job was unaware of such a discussion. (It was divine classified information.) But then, we are not privy to the heavenly discussions about us either. Like Job though, *how* we walk through the mysteries of life when we don't know and we can't understand, is of profound significance.

CHAPTER TWENTY-ONE

One Crisis after Another

The theatre curtain comes down on the heavenly chambers and the scene changes dramatically. Drums can be heard rumbling in the distance as the curtain rises again, indicating that foreboding storm clouds are building over Job's family. Serenity is about to give way to calamity. Nothing could ever have prepared Job for this. He had no premonitions or prior warnings that we know of. One day everything was sweet. The next day everything turned sour.

Job's sons and daughters were feasting at their older brother's house. The oxen were plowing and the donkeys were grazing in the fields as usual, when neighboring enemies attacked without warning and stole the cattle. Then they killed the servants. Only one escaped, and he ran to deliver the terrible message to Job. Even while he was speaking, another messenger rushed in gasping for breath, telling of more trouble; "The fire of God fell from the sky and burned up the sheep and the servants, and I am the only one who has escaped to tell you!" Eugene Peterson descriptively paraphrases this verse in *The Message;* "Bolts of lightning struck the sheep and the shepherds and fried them – burned them to a crisp." This was not a good day at the office!

Job had just gone bankrupt! His food stocks and shares simply plummeted to zero! His mind was still reeling, when another scared servant burst through the door with news of a different catastrophe; "The Chaldeans formed three raiding parties and swept down on your camels and carried them off. They also killed the servants." All Job's servants have been massacred in one day (except for the three that got away), and his livelihood has been totally decimated. How is he going to tell his wife?

However, nothing could have prepared him for the next bearer of bad news. This was the worst shock of all. "A mighty wind swept in from the desert and struck the four corners of the house where your sons and daughters were feasting. It collapsed on them and they are dead." His children are dead! *All* of them! Ten new coffins needed. Ten fresh graves to be dug. Not just one killed. Not two or three. Not seven or eight, but ten! As their father, he had regularly prayed that the Lord would protect each one. Now they are all gone in one powerful tornado. There are no words in the dictionary that can even come close to describing the magnitude of Job's heart pain

162

in that moment. And how does his wife deal with this? A mother's heart is left barren and broken!

Satan is so cruel. As soon as he had God's permission, he was gone in a flash, to carry out his venomous intent. In one day, Job's family, finances, food and servants had been wiped out!

I remember when Len and I were in Malaysia, preaching at a church conference. It was held in the lofty Genting Highlands. The magnificent retreat was so high up in the mountains, that often the clouds hovered at the revolving front door and literally squeezed their way into the large entrance hall. On the top level of this classy hotel was the casino gaming floor. People saved up their money and would then spend the weekend, gambling away their hard-earned cash. Some left walking on air. Others left in coffins!

Even while we were staying there, a terrible commotion broke out. Someone, we were told, had just jumped to his death, having lost all his life-savings at the gambling table. The air was thick with devastation. People crying. Reality biting hard. Everything gone. He had no reason to live anymore. So he didn't. His money crashed. So did he, on the hard concrete floor of the mountain get-away. What a tragic end!

Job knew these emotions; the shock, the horror and the brutal torment of gut-wrenching losses. Nevertheless, his response is even more remarkable. The unknown man in our previous story jumped to his death because life became meaningless for him the moment he lost his money. Yet, here in stark contrast, we see Job rising to

163

his feet. He takes his robe, tears it and shaves his head. What is he doing? Is he angry? Perhaps he's lost it? No, surprisingly he hasn't. It seems a strange thing to do nowadays but at that time, these were symbols for mourning, signs of loss and evidence of deep grief. Job falls to the ground, but thankfully, not from the thirteenth floor of a casino building. Then he worships! There's no drum roll or music, no heavenly choir to move his emotions. He just bows his heart and praises God.

How extraordinary! Listen to the cry of a man who, although he can hardly find words to describe what has just happened to him, begins to pour out his heart to God; "The Lord gave and the Lord has taken away; may the name of the Lord be praised." What a man!

Job doesn't blame anyone. He doesn't accuse his servants for not defending his cattle or chasing away the marauders. He doesn't curse God for the lightning strike or the deadly tornado. He doesn't rail on God and ask why He didn't stop the destructive forces that have just devastated his family. He doesn't rant and rave and throw things at anyone. Job just gives himself permission to grieve in the best way he knows. He glorifies God, recognizing His sovereignty in this horrific drama. He'd been given so much. Now it was gone. He mourns but is not angry. He doesn't sin by charging God with any wrongdoing. Incredible!

Genuine trust is a rare treasure, like gold mined from the secret places in the earth. Believing that God's purposes are good, even if circumstances seem to scream the opposite, brings great praise and honor to God. It's a radiant quality that sparkles from a life that has gone through the purifying flames, and learned to thank the divine hands that stoked the refiner's fire!

The great 19th century preacher, Charles Spurgeon and his wife Susannah, knew what it was to suffer severely. The words, "I have chosen thee in the furnace of affliction" (from Isaiah 48:10), were strategically placed on their bedroom wall. They were also inscribed on their hearts! In his daily devotional, '*Faith's Checkbook*,' Spurgeon writes, 'We are chosen…not in the palace but in the furnace. In the furnace, beauty is marred, fashion is destroyed, strength is melted, glory is consumed; yet eternal love reveals its secrets, and declares its choice. So has it been in our case…Therefore, if the furnace be heated seven times hotter, we will not dread it, for the glorious Son of God will walk with us amid the glowing coals.'

Susannah later recorded the memory of an incident when this also became a revelation to her. In the early years of their marriage, she had been intensely involved in the life of their church. She often accompanied Charles on his travels whenever it was possible. But when she was 36, like an eagle in full flight, she was struck down by a serious health condition that often left her bed-ridden for lengthy periods of time. Her wings remained clipped for the rest of her life! Loneliness and isolation became unwelcome intruders in her home. She says, "For many years, I was a prisoner in a sick chamber." Only the memories of her previous active lifestyle were eventually left to remind her of her many losses. This was to be an enduring sadness and a heavy yoke that both husband and wife graciously shouldered together.

After one of these long periods of illness, Susannah wrote of one particular Sunday evening. Her husband was away preaching at the Metropolitan Tabernacle, and she had stayed home with a friend who was keeping her company. As evening fell towards the end of a dark and dismal day, she felt as if some of the outside darkness seemed to have entered her own soul. Doubts, like hungry vultures, fed on her despair. She was depressed, and with a sorrowful heart she asked, "Why does my Lord God so often send sharp and bitter pain to visit me? Why does my Lord thus deal with His child?"

Her questions were answered in the form of a parable. It was a cold night and the fire was burning. All was quiet for a while, when suddenly she was surprised by a sound from deep within one of the logs. Susannah recorded her amazement;

"We listened again and heard the faint plaintive notes, so sweet, so melodious, yet mysterious enough to provoke for a moment our undisguised wonder…It was as though the fire was letting loose the imprisoned music from the old oaks' innermost heart. A song from the fire!" She quickly drew the parallel; "Ah, I thought, when the fire of affliction draws songs of praise from us, then indeed are we purified and our God is glorified. Perhaps some of us are like this old oak log…we should give forth no melodious sounds were it not for the fire which kindles round us and releases tender notes of trust in Him and cheerful compliance to His will…Singing in the fire!

Yes! God helping us, if that is the only way to get harmony out of these hard apathetic hearts, let the furnace be heated seven times hotter than before." (Charles Ray *Mrs. C.H. Spurgeon.*)

What a woman! What worship in the midst of adversity! Praise burns up our questions, leaves our doubts in the ashes and lifts our spirits above the embers of pain. Why would we blame God for the tragedies in our lives? God cannot do evil. He is pure and holy. The Psalmist says, 'God is good to all and His tender mercies are over all His works (Psalm 145:9 NKJV).

Therefore, in the light of this, how do we process a story like Job's? God clearly allowed Satan to do his worst, but God didn't do wrong. (There are certain things God could prevent by His power, that He may permit in His wisdom.) He could have thwarted every single one of these disasters, but He didn't. God allowed the testing of one of his favorite friends, for His own good and perfect reasons. He also knew how much He was going to bless him later. However, Job had no inkling of this. For all he knew, his life as he'd known it was over, and that was it.

There is an amazing verse in Ephesians 3:10. It says that 'now, through the church, the manifold (i.e. many-sided as the facets of a diamond) wisdom of God should be made known to the rulers and authorities in the heavenly realms.' What is God revealing? His great wisdom. To whom is He displaying it? The unseen heavenly host. Who is He using as the diamonds to reflect His glory? You and me!

If ever there was a man who reflected the glory of God, it was Job in this moment of worship. If ever there is someone who displays the marvelous wisdom of God to myriads of invisible principalities, it is the child of God who falls before the Lord in loving reverence and adoration, even when they don't understand the reasons for the trials they are facing.

My son Matt tells of an experience one time when he was lying lifeless on our lounge room floor. He was so weak he could barely move. His strength had gone and his legs felt as heavy as concrete. Everyone has a breaking point – an inner elastic band that can only stretch so far. Matt's resolve seemed as if it was about to break. For the first time in six years, he found himself wanting to ask God the question, "Why?" But before he had even finished formulating the word in his mind, he heard God lovingly, yet so clearly say, "You're asking the wrong question!" Now this was quite some statement from God! And unexpected!

After a few speechless moments, Matt thought, "Well, what is the right question?" Immediately, he heard God say, "Can you trust Me, no matter what?" Just seven small words! However, the impact was huge. As he pondered the gravity of this question, Matt hung scarily suspended in the mid-air of uncertainty. There were really only two choices; "Yes" or "No!" But how do you say "No" to an all-perfect, all-merciful and all-loving God? What would it mean though, if he said "Yes" and what might that involve?

After searching his heart for some time, while trying to avoid the implications of his reply, Matt felt ready to say, "Yes I can!" But halfway through answering, he was caught by the awareness of an even greater gravity. Then he realized, "No I can't! I need *Your help* Lord, to trust You no matter what!"

This was an incredibly significant and timely encounter. From that moment, everything changed. It was as if God picked Matt up and held him in His arms in the most remarkable way. Dependence on the Lord always brings new hope and strength. It has for Matt, even in the darkest of days during the long struggle that has lasted well over 12 years!

The bottom line has always been trust, even when we do not and cannot understand. Will we still praise and thank God when we are under the most intense pressure? Worship displays His infinite wisdom and love to thousands of invisible spectators. Angels watch in wonder. Demons watch too. Not with wonder but rampant envy, as we glorify God through our trials. How fragrant is the aroma of the sacrifice of praise!

It always is!

CHAPTER TWENTY-TWO

But Wait, There's More!

However, Job's trial isn't over yet! Satan still hasn't vented his final fury upon God's friend. In Job chapter 2, we find that this fiendish creature has the audacity to attend yet another of these heavenly meetings where God is talking to His angels. Once again, God turns to Satan and asks him where he has been. He gives the same answer as before; roaming throughout the earth, and watching everything that's going on. Same old, same old. Nothing's new.

The Lord still has Job on His mind. "Have you considered my servant, how amazing he is? Have you noticed that he is still keeping his integrity through all the pain you've inflicted on him?" Job has indeed been severely tried, but has come forth shining as pure gold. Satan skeptically replies, "A man will give all he has for his own life.

But stretch out your hand and strike his flesh and bones, and he will surely curse you to your face."

"Very well then," the Lord replies, "he's in your hands but you must spare his life." Divine consent is granted. Satan does not need to be given permission twice. The boundary is clear but he can work around that. His pernicious plans have already been conceived.

In the blink of an eye he is gone, rubbing his demonic hands with glee. He knows how to hurt Job, even if he can't destroy him. Painful stinging sores, searing like hot irons all through the day and night. Stinging and itchy scabs from the top of his head to the soles of his feet, that only broken bits of pottery can help relieve. Physical agony! That will get him cursing the God he claims to serve.

How hungry is Satan to hear the first bitter words from Job's lips toward God! He's hungry to hear us cursing God too! Then he has won the battle. Our last lifeline of fellowship with God will have been broken. Satan had that intimacy once, but he won't ever know the joy of that friendship again. His wants to make sure you don't have it either! So he'll try everything in his power to make you bitter. You'll recognize his goading spur; "Blame God, go on!" He knows that if you do, from that moment on you will feel very alone. Satan's work will be done. He can then sit back, rubbing those same hands with demonic delight. Another one bites the dust!

Even now, you might be going through a most traumatic time in your life, whether it be physical affliction, emotional stress or a spiritual trial. You may have lost everything. Your husband or wife could be in the process of leaving you. Your son or daughter may have been diagnosed with a chronic or terminal illness. Perhaps you are under more pressure than you can bear. Trapped in a situation, seemingly without solutions, you are wondering if God even cares about you, let alone feels your pain. Satan would love you to doubt God. It's exactly what he's counting on!

Your Heavenly Father doesn't allow you to suffer lightly. God loves you. In Lamentations 3:33 we read, "If He works severely, He also works tenderly. His stockpiles of loyal love are immense. He takes no pleasure in making life hard, in throwing roadblocks in the way" (*The Message*). Every single loss you endure is absorbed by the heart of God. He sees every tear you cry.

My husband Len wrote a song a few years ago entitled, *'Don't Doubt His Love.'* It shows that because God has suffered more than we'll ever comprehend, He cares more than we'll ever understand!

You've suffered; times you've wondered why,
Even thought that God had passed you by.
You've wondered, is this what loves planned
Does He care, does He understand?

He suffered more than any man,
Broke His heart so you would understand.
He's traveled the depths of your despair;
Every road leads to His heart of care.

173

His body was marred, as sin left its brands.

They drove great spikes through His feet and His hands.

His spirit was crushed, His soul tasted hell.

The pain He bore no tongue can tell.

The sun turned to night, the Father turned away.

Fists and spit let the world have its say.

Desperate tides of a whole world's pain

Forced their way through every vein.

Your sorrow's not worthy to compare

With all the weight of glory you will share.

You'll see Him, the Lamb, the Lion, the Dove,

And wonder how you doubted such great love.

Don't doubt His love

Don't doubt His love.

Do *not* doubt His love! Sure, Job questioned it at times, but he never stopped trusting God, even in the darkest of days. However, when Job needed his wife's help the most, her only encouragement and advice was to give up! "Why don't you just curse God and die?" No doubt, she was also in great pain. She'd attended the funerals of her children. She'd lost her livelihood, her future, and her husband didn't seem to be the same anymore. Had she even lost her faith?

Life certainly hadn't turned out the way she'd expected. Dreams for her family had been shattered by her losses as well. Disappointment and pain can often turn ugly.

It's not hard to be bitter. Neither is it difficult to grow weeds. Those pesky plants seem to grow anywhere and everywhere, even between the tiniest of cracks. Far more care is required to cultivate flowers. It doesn't take much to mouth off at your husband or wife when you're under the pump. How much better to have God's love and grace growing in your life, so you can give that same gentleness and understanding to those you love when they need your support. A soft answer and a loving touch means so much to those who are hurting. It's a tangible gift wrapped up with your own life that says, "I love you."

Job's wife was unable to give such a gift to her husband in his time of need. Her faith had been too badly shaken. Her sorrow was too great! Job chose to worship. She didn't. Grief can express itself in many different ways. How precious it is when pain is processed through praise and worship. The incense from this costly sacrifice is undeniably sweet. It's the instantly recognizable fragrance of love under pressure and grace under fire. Job's response was not angry but measured; "Shall we accept only good things from the hand of God, and never anything bad?" What a piecing question!

David says in Psalm 119:68, 'You are *good* and what You do is *good.*' However, just three verses later he says, 'It was *good* for me to be afflicted so that I might learn Your decrees.' There is an intrinsic connection here. The outworking of what God knows is best for us may well include some trouble, but it will always be good!

The apostle Paul had 'trouble!' He had a persistent problem he described as a 'thorn in his flesh.' We're not told exactly what it was, but it was a big enough irritation for him to ask God three times to remove it from him, but each time the answer was a resolute "No!" Why was this? Because Paul was being punished? Because his faith wasn't strong enough? Not at all! God firmly but gently reassured him, "My grace is sufficient for you, for My power is made perfect in weakness" (2 Corinthians 12:9).

Here was a perfect opportunity for God to display His power and strength in whatever frustration Paul was experiencing. But the 'thorn' had an important purpose and therefore needed to remain. It would prevent him from becoming proud and keep him humbly dependent on God's grace as he shared that same grace with others. What incredible peace comes when we bow before God's wisdom. At this point our theology of suffering has begun.

Charles Spurgeon told of a time when he was riding home after a heavy day's work. He was exhausted and depressed. Suddenly, he remembered the promise, "My grace is sufficient for you." After he reached home and examined the original text, he laughed to himself. It made unbelief seem so absurd. It was as though some thirsty little fish was troubled about drinking the river dry, when it heard the invitation, "Drink away little fish, my stream is sufficient for you." So it is with God's grace. Like a mighty ocean, it will never run dry!

Grace! The measureless kindness and favor of God expressing itself freely in unlimited love. What a spectacular word! Spurgeon encouraged his hearers to be great believers. "Little faith will bring your souls to heaven but great faith will bring heaven to your souls." He made the point so simply, yet succinctly: God might not always remove the irritating and painful thorn, but He has an inexhaustible supply of grace to strengthen and comfort us, and even bless us in our troubles.

Job's friends

Job had a few 'thorns' to endure. The dictionary definition of a thorn is: 'A small sharp-pointed tip resembling a spike on a stem or leaf. A prickle. Something that causes irritation and annoyance.' (Colloquially used, it can mean: A nuisance. A pain in the neck!)

Job's three thorns came cleverly disguised as friends. They had heard of Job's afflictions, so they came to give their support. If only they hadn't opened their mouths! One of the dearest comforts you can have when you are really suffering are your closest friends. True friends say kind things to your face *and* behind your back. They are one in a million. (I remember when Len said that about me once to a member of our congregation, "My wife's one in a million!" Our friend replied, "Oh really? My wife was won in a raffle." Sorry!)

I have already mentioned how precious my friends were during my journey with cancer. Many came with meals when I was just too sick to cook. Other paid the fees for my radiation treatments, some drove me to and from the hospital. Rosters were drawn up because so many wanted to help. A holiday was organized and paid for so that Len and I could just escape and get away for a few days. To all my wonderful friends, and you know who you are, words alone will never adequately express how much I treasure you. You brought us such comfort by your acts of kindness, that helped to sweeten our bitter trials.

However, Job didn't have such treasures. His so-called friends brought him confrontation instead of comfort, accusation instead of consolation. Understandably, they must have been devastated to see him covered with sores, sitting on a rubbish dump, but why had such tragedy happened to him?

Before long, they had it all worked out. Off they went on their tiresome tirades and their bleak theories of why he was in such a terrible predicament. Surely, Job must have brought this on himself. It was his fault. He was to blame. Together they held their torches of incrimination, shining the spotlight of their judgments upon his misery and failure. The hurt and disappointment he expressed was well-justified; "One should be kind to a fainting friend, but you have accused me without the slightest fear of the Almighty…You have proved as unreliable as a seasonal brook that overflows its bank in the spring when it is swollen with ice and melting snow. But when the hot weather arrives, the water disappears."

How sad! These men had brought an altogether different kind of anguish. Misguided friends, whose silver-forked tongues hissed out words filled with poison. Job's pain was palpable: "The caravans turn aside to be refreshed, but there is nothing to drink, and so they perish in the desert...their hopes are dashed. You too have proved to be of no help" (Job 6:14-20 NLT).

What heartless cruelty he had to endure. He is confounded but doesn't conceal his frustration and disappointment: "How long will you torment me and crush me with your words? Ten times now you have reproached me; shamelessly you attack me...All my intimate friends detest me; those I love have turned against me" (Job 19:1-3 and 19). There's no natural antidote for heartache like this!

God was angry with Job's friends, as they had made inferences about Him that were not true. The man they condemned was God's friend! They were in serious trouble! (No wonder they were told to humble themselves before Job, so he could sacrifice burnt offerings on their behalf, and pray for them! They needed serious help!)

We can be very vulnerable during times of extreme stress. It is so easy to be misjudged and misrepresented. Some people you think would care, stay away because they just don't know what to do or say. However, that is preferable to those who think they know what you are going through and try to help, but end up making hurtful remarks that leave you feeling totally misunderstood.

The greatest gift you can give is understanding. Hurting people don't need answers as much as they long to feel the healing balm of unconditional love. It's like soothing ointment on a wounded soul. Pour it out in generous portions. You'll never lack friends if you do!

Job's consternation – God's revelation

Understandably, there were moments when Job's endurance teetered precariously on the precipice of his limited understanding. He looked back longingly to his halcyon days. He could remember when his family was living under the canopy of God's blessing, and surrounded by that wonderful hedge of protection. The days when he still had his children and everything he touched turned to gold! Nothing was even remotely clear as to why everything had changed so suddenly. Would there ever be any relief for his pain?

One day, while Job was musing, the sky darkened and ominous clouds began to gather around his house. Rain splattered against the windows. Thunder grumbled in the background. Lightning flashed incessantly. Howling winds moaned in a foreboding tone. From the midst of this violent storm, God spoke. With the authority of divine majesty, His words dropped like hailstones into Job's heart.

"Why do you talk without knowing what you're talking about? I have some questions for you. Where were you when I created the earth? Who decided on its size? Who came up with the blueprints and measurements? How was its foundation poured and who set the cornerstone, while the morning stars sang in chorus and all the angels shouted praise? And who took charge of the ocean when it gushed forth like a baby from the womb? Do you know where Light comes from and where Darkness lives? Have you ever traveled to where the snow is made, and seen the vault where hail is stockpiled? Can you find your way to where lightning is launched or to the place from which the wind blows? Can you take charge of the lightning bolts and have then report to you for orders?

God's questions continued, cascading like rivers from heaven. "Now what do you have to say for yourself? Are you going to haul Me, the Mighty One, into court and press charges?" Job was left shell-shocked and silent! Not one further complaint passed his lips. Just the repentant words, "I'm speechless, in awe – words fail me. I should never have opened my mouth...I've talked too much. I'm sorry – forgive me. I'll never do that again, I promise! I'll never live again on crusts of hearsay, crumbs of rumor" (see Job 38–42 *The Message*). He was so very sorry!

How could he argue anymore? Then why should we, when we have questions? Does the clay complain to the Potter if the grip of His hand seems too firm? Can the creature advise the Creator about the designs of His creations?

When we don't understand, the best thing to do is what Job did. Realize how big God is and how small we are. Then just trust in His faithful love and worship!

CHAPTER TWENTY-THREE

The Grand Finale

God causes 'all things to work together for good.' What an amazing promise. But, it doesn't apply to everyone! It's *only* for those 'who love God and ...are called according to His purpose' (Romans 8:28 NASB). Job loved God. However, it certainly didn't seem as though everything was working out for good. His suffering was epic, but he never lost hope. Incredibly, he was still able to say, "Though He slay me, *yet* will I trust in Him" (Job 13:15 KJV).

Pain can leave a lasting imprint on the ones who have had to endure it. We may never be the same again. Neither will our families who have weathered the storms with us. Either we will emerge from our trials, bitter or better; traumatized by our trials, or transformed by God's power, grateful for its life-changing impact.

James, the brother of Jesus, uses Job as a classic example of long-suffering, whilst encouraging us not to despair in our trials. He says, "You have heard of Job's perseverance and have seen what the Lord finally brought about. The Lord is full of compassion and mercy" (James 5:11). This tells us what God loved about his friend; his patient endurance under the most unbelievable pressure, even when he couldn't understand. It also shows us what we love about God; His heart that is full of compassion. ('Full!' meaning abundant, bursting, brimming, copious, complete, unconditional, all-inclusive, all-encompassing and unrestricted. It's as deep as the oceans and as high as the heavens!) The loving heart that is behind all our trials, is also unfathomably wise.

Did Job behave impeccably throughout his trials? *No!* Did he curse the day he was born? *Yes!* Was God punishing him? *No!* Did He bless him anyway? *Yes!* Why? Because God is so gracious.

Amazingly, Job and his wife stayed together through it all! That was a miracle. Most marriages would have crumbled in a heap under such pressure. Marriages *can* be restored and love *can* blossom again. Two hearts *can* survive the savage seas if there is unconditional love and patient understanding.

Yes, traumatic things did happen to Job, but his life doesn't end in a melancholic minor key. Ecclesiastes 3 says, 'There is a time for everything; a time to weep and a time to laugh, a time to mourn and a time to dance.' Finally, the time came for Job's celebration! It's as if vibrant major chords resound from the heavenly orchestra, directed by the divine conductor and the joyful intensity culminates in a rising crescendo of crashing cymbals. God hadn't forgotten His friend! He had always known what the Grand Finale would look like. It was impressive!

Feasting was an important priority in Job's household. So after his trials were over, his brothers and sisters and everyone else who had known him previously, came and joined the festivities. I'm sure they ate and drank with absolute abandon. (Well, someone had to continue the family tradition!) It's interesting that they came at the end of his trauma! How much better to have known their love and encouragement in the tough times! But at least they knew what to bring to the party: 'Each one gave him a piece of silver and a gold ring!' (Good call!) They 'comforted and consoled him over all the trouble the Lord had brought upon him' (Job 42:11).

Does God allow trouble? Apparently so! However, we read of the extraordinary conclusion in Job 42; 'After Job had prayed for his friends, the Lord made him prosperous again and gave him twice as much as he had before…The Lord blessed the latter part of Job's life more than the first.' He received double the number of sheep, camels, oxen and donkeys. He had ten more children; seven boys and three stunningly beautiful girls. He lived life to the fullest for another 140 years. His children married and they had their own families Job lived to see four generations of grandkids. He sure hit the finish line running! Never could he have begun to imagine the wonderful future God had planned for him.

Neither can we! The apostle Paul writes, 'No eye has seen, no ear has heard, no mind has conceived what God has prepared for those who love Him' (1 Corinthians 2:9). Did Job ever envisage that his life would be so sweet and satisfying in his latter years. He must have experienced blessings he never thought were even remotely possible.

Job's experience is an amazing example of 'patience in the face of suffering.' Thankfully, our situations aren't all as extreme as his. But we all have Job's God! He can turn our trials into triumphs and our sorrows into joy. Nature paints the picture: When the tide ebbs to its lowest point, it turns to rise again; when winter is over, spring appears and new shoots bud again; when night has almost gone, the darkness gives way to soft rays of dawn, bringing fresh hope for a new day. We may not sink to the depths of Job's poverty or rise to the heights of his wealth, but the same loving God who turned Job's captivity into such blessing, can bring about a turning point for us as well.

What an extraordinary ending to such a horrendously painful story. All the time, God was silently working in the shadows of Job's afflictions, planning to bless him in the most unbelievable way. And so He is with us!

CHAPTER TWENTY-FOUR

Can Any Good Come from Suffering?

What good can possibly come out of pain? It helps to know, because few experiences are more universal than suffering. When I'm hurting, I need faith to see beyond my circumstances, to the divine purpose behind it all. God loves us and longs to bless us. He knows what is ultimately best for us. Will we trust Him?

In the Old Testament, blessings from God were dependent on His people's obedience. Deuteronomy 28 gives a comprehensive list of God's requirements; *If* they obeyed the Lord and carefully followed all His commands, then blessings would come upon them. They would be blessed in the city and blessed in the country. Their children would be blessed, as would their crops and animals. They would be blessed when they went in and when they went out. Their enemies would be defeated before them. Everything they put their hand to would be blessed. On and on the blessings continued, but they were all conditional. The problem was the big *'If'* right at the start. They couldn't possibly fulfill the conditions. Ever!

Neither can we, which is why Jesus came. He kept the Law and fulfilled its exacting demands. When Jesus died on the cross He paid our penalty for breaking the Law (with its impossible requirements and frightening consequences), so God could bless unconditionally and perfectly justly. Now, those who have put their faith in Him are in the new covenant which is not based on keeping rules but on a relationship with God.

At the Last Supper, when Jesus offered His disciples a cup of wine, He explained it represented the 'blood of the new covenant, which is poured out for many for the forgiveness of sins' (Matthew 26:28). We are not bound by the old covenant anymore. The new one has come. We have been forgiven! 1 John 3:1 says, 'How great is the love the Father has lavished on us, that we should be called children of God!' How amazing that we should be objects of such extravagant love!

Now we are in God's new covenant, our blessings are not only in this world. They are also spiritual. We have been blessed 'in the heavenly realms with every spiritual blessing in Christ' (Ephesians 1:3). Our earthly blessings are temporary. Our spiritual blessings are treasures forever. God promises that our pain and sorrows are all going to be worth it. How can this be and in what way?

1) We're going to share in God's glory!

We have been guaranteed of something far more enduring than material blessings. We are being prepared to share the glory of God. The apostle Paul explains in 2 Corinthians 4:17-18 (AMP), 'For our light, momentary affliction (this slight distress of the passing hour) is ever more and more abundantly preparing and producing and achieving for us an everlasting weight of glory [beyond all measure, excessively surpassing all comparisons and all calculations, a vast and transcendent glory and blessedness never to cease!]'

In his book *Suffering and the Sovereignty of God,* John Piper points out that Paul didn't just endure his trials because of his great hope in heaven. He knew that his afflictions were preparing him for glory, and these sufferings would have a direct effect on the weight of that glory. 'For I consider that the sufferings of this present time are not worthy to be compared with the glory that is to be revealed in us' (Romans 8:18 NASB).

Paul knew exactly what he was talking about because he had suffered so greatly. He is not ashamed. In fact, he boasts about what he had been through. He had been in prison frequently and flogged severely. He had been whipped, stoned, beaten with rods, and had faced death repeatedly. He had been shipwrecked several times. He had been at risk from rivers, threatened by robbers, betrayed by his own people and opposed by the Gentiles. He had known perils in the city, dangers in the deserts and exposure in the open seas. He had lived with weariness and pain, gone without sleep, been hungry and thirsty, cold and naked. Then, added to all this, he had the daily pressure of caring for all the churches (see 2 Corinthians 11: 23-28). What a list of his excruciating distresses; spiritually, physically and emotionally. But, as Paul looks back, he considers them 'slight and momentary' in comparison to the weight of glory that is coming!

My heart thrills as I write these words. This gives me purpose in my pain. This is the inspiration that enables me to persevere. This encourages me to rejoice, even when my heart is breaking under a heavy weight of sorrow. One day I'm going to exchange it for a far greater weight – of glory! What an incredible relief when the burden of pain will be lifted and replaced with the crown of life.

Sharing in God's glory, however, is not automatic. We qualify "*if*" we share in His sufferings (Romans 8:17). So perhaps we should even consider it a blessing!

2) We're being prepared to reign with Christ

When we understand the purpose of suffering, we will see our trials and suffering as a privilege. God is not punishing us for our sins. Jesus satisfied God's wrath for sin in offering Himself as our perfect sacrifice, once and for all. God is planning to bless us more than we can ever imagine. 'And since we are His children, we will share His treasures – for everything God gives to His Son, Christ, is ours too. But, if we are to share His glory, we must also share His suffering' (Romans 8:17 NLT). 'If we endure, we will also reign with Him' (2 Timothy 2:12). This is not punitive! This is training for reigning with Christ one day! In the light of this, our trials take on a wonderful new meaning. God has a specific purpose in allowing everything we go through.

The apostle Peter explains what is happening to us; '...though now for a little while you may have had to suffer grief in all kinds of trials. These have come so that your faith–of greater worth than gold, which perishes even though refined by fire–may be proved genuine and may result in praise, glory and honor when Jesus Christ is revealed' (1 Peter 1:6-7).

When it comes to having an understanding of suffering, these are vital and significant scriptures. They help us to endure joyfully, and fill us with hope. 'Weeping may endure (literally meaning 'lodge as a guest') for a night, but joy comes in the morning' (Psalm 30:5 NKJV). Weeping is the natural overflow of a heart that is breaking and sometimes the night season can seem eternally long, but joy will come. Pain is extremely unpleasant. It may well leave a tart taste in our soul. But when we trust God, He can take the bitter experiences and make them sweet. Then the metamorphosis has begun and the transformation is on its way.

God knows what is required to bring this about. We don't just wake up one day, jump out of bed and suddenly discover we have a theology of suffering. This can only be forged in the fiery furnace of intense pressure.

However, the change that eventually takes place in our lives is well worth it. God thinks so!

John and Tracey's story

I was talking recently to my friend John. He's a neighbor living in our street, whose family we have come to love and respect. The first time I met them was at a 'neighborhood watch' family day held at our park, just across the road. Tracey, his wife, was wheeling a pushchair. Nothing strange about that, except in it was their autistic nine-year-old son, Rowan. He can't walk many steps without being physically supported. His head drops over to one side, his eyes dart searchingly and his hands flail uncontrollably.

How much does he understand? Will he ever be able to tell us? Not at the moment, anyway. Nevertheless, Tracey and John shower him with devotion and love him unconditionally. They cherish and protect him in every way possible. His disabilities don't change their commitment to care for him. They are such an inspiration to me.

As John and I were talking, we were sharing about the weight of pain that we as parents carry for our children, especially when we watch them suffer and there is nothing we can do about it. He made the comment, "It's like a dull ache that just won't go away." I knew exactly what he meant.

What would it be like to be a normal family? Carefree and full of fun, without the constant adrenaline rush of intense sorrow and stress. For some of us, it's how we live and we've almost forgotten the feeling of freedom that comes when living without tragedy.

With the benefit of hindsight, would John and Tracey still have chosen to have Rowan? I know they would! He is such a joy to them and they love him so much. There's no way they would give him back! They are the best parents he could have. They have embraced their life together with dignity, grace, and even laughter! They stand as a shining beacon in our community.

Would they be the amazing people they are today if they hadn't gone through their trials associated with autism? Who knows? But I'm sure it's the pressure they have endured that has made them the priceless jewels they are. They might not see themselves as we do, and probably have no idea what an encouragement they are. It's like that with suffering. Others draw strength from us, although we are not even aware that anyone is watching.

There is indeed purpose in our pain!

CHAPTER TWENTY-FIVE

Pain, the Carpenter's Chisel

When we were originally created, God made us in His image. But when sin entered our world, we became self-centered and our likeness to God was marred. However, In Ezekiel 36:26, God says, 'I will give you a new heart and put a new spirit in you; I will remove from you your heart of stone and give you a heart of flesh. And I will put my Spirit in you...' God has work to do!

Paul explains that when we belong to God, He starts the huge task of conforming us to the likeness of His Son (see Romans 8:29). Purposefully, He takes His chisel in one hand and our heart in the other. Then skillfully, He cuts into the crevices of our lives, carving carefully and deliberately, until the resemblance of Jesus begins to appear. Unfortunately, this doesn't just happen automatically. Pain and suffering are the very tools required to etch into our hearts for that change to take place.

They were for King David. Yet, in David's early life, he would never have guessed the way in which God was going transform him. He was the youngest of eight and the least in his father's house. His chores were far away in the fields, caring for sheep; certainly not the most illustrious job. In the lonely pastures, he played his harp and sang his psalms, as he whiled away the hours.

Therefore, he would have been quite startled one day, to see a servant running towards him. Rarely anyone came over to his office on the hills. What was the occasion? Maybe he was trouble!

"Your father wants you straight away!" Surely, that was a red warning light, right there! The fact that the prophet Samuel was at the house waiting for him wasn't a good sign either. Perhaps he was in trouble with God! When David breathlessly fell in the door, he would have been amazed to see everyone standing, waiting for him to arrive! The atmosphere was electric! What was going on?

Samuel knew the Lord had spoken to him about anointing one of these brothers to be the next king on Israel's throne. But which one? He'd already seen the other seven, and none of them had been God's choice. Immediately the prophet laid eyes on Jesse's youngest son, the Lord's definitive "Yes," resonated in his heart. "Rise and anoint him. *He* is the one."

Right then and there, in front of his dad and bewildered older brothers, David was singled out and anointed to be king. From that day, the Spirit of the Lord powerfully came upon him. Chosen by God, David would ultimately rise from total obscurity, to the most prestigious and influential position in his country. King of Israel!

At least there would be no more rescuing sheep from a myriad of potholes. No more shearing and removing burs from their wool. No more searching for pasture and staying awake all night guarding his sheep from marauding beasts. No more wrestling with lions and bears. Great! When would the coronation be?

Not so fast David! Not nearly so fast. There is much work to do first. The carpenter's chisel has to carve your heart into a kingly shape. Some suffering will be necessary. People will be jealous of you. Enemies will come against you. You will be tempted to retaliate but patience will be forged into your spirit in the fires of adversity. If you are going to lead My people, you will have to learn to trust Me as your God. My ways are not your ways David. I am going to make you into a man after My own heart. However, it won't happen overnight. Shaping and chiseling take time but, it will be well worth it. Wait and see!

Wait? Did he hear the word "wait"? Not verbally, not literally, though his experience would bear it out. Training for reigning takes time. Troubles and distresses are inevitable. Like what? Like being afraid for his life. Experiencing betrayal. Losing his child, his home, his best friend, his throne, his confidence and self-respect! Living in a dark and dingy cave, with no food and security, no hope, and seemingly no future.

Oh, and did we forget to mention it would mean fighting with giants? What? Don't kings live in magnificent palaces? Aren't they given preferential treatment to prepare them for impressive official duties? Don't people bow before their thrones? Don't guards stand to attention and salute them because they're all-important now?

Samuel did not mention any of this to David, as he anointed him to be king! Neither does God tell us all we must endure as the Carpenter chisels a cross-shape into our lives. Apparently, there's much cutting and chipping that's required!

When David looked back over the years, he remembered how God had saved him many times. He'd gone through some severe trials. So had the nation he served. But these were all an essential part of their spectacular deliverance!

"Praise our God…
He has preserved our lives
and kept our feet from slipping.
For You Oh God, tested us;
You refined us like silver.
You brought us into prison
and laid burdens on our backs.
You let men ride over our heads;
we went through fire and water,
But, you brought us (out) to a place of abundance."
(Psalm 66:8-12)

This is not David thanking God for setting him free *from* his suffering. He is glorying in the fact that God has blessed him *in and through* his suffering. You have 'enlarged me when I was in distress!' (Psalm 4:1 KJV). God is expanding David's heart, exchanging a lean spirit for a fat one!

Notice the phrases that David uses in Psalm 66 to describe the chisel's work in his life: 'Tested…refined…brought us into prison …laid burdens on us…let men ride over our heads…went through fire and water!' These words convey indications of some significant carvings! Here we have the process that is involved, and the result at the end. Thankfully we read the word '*but*' after all of this. God is bringing us out to a place of 'abundance' which means 'lushness, luxuriance, overflow, plenty, profusion, richness, and wealth.' What a wonderful word! However, if we are being shaped into the image of God's Son, the chisel must be applied. So, is there a purpose in our pain? Is all the suffering worth it? You be the judge!

Personally, it helps me to know the answer to these questions if I am going to run the race and finish well! It's not difficult to start running with an initial burst of energy, but what happens if I fall over, or clip the hurdle and tumble onto the gritty concrete? Will I give up and collapse in a crumpled heap, weeping for what might have been, or will I pick myself up and brush myself down, knowing that God is strengthening me and willing me on?

Eugene Peterson paraphrases 1 Corinthians 9:24-25, 'You've all been to the stadium and seen the athletes race. Everyone runs;

one wins. All good athletes train hard. They do it for a gold medal that tarnishes and fades. You're after the one that's gold eternally.' He then continues 'I don't know about you, but I'm running hard for the finishing line. I'm giving it everything I've got' (*The Message*). Maybe I won't be the fastest runner. Maybe I won't get first prize. But, there is a rich reward for finishing well. In James 1:12, 'Blessed is the man who perseveres under trial, because when he has stood the test, he will receive the crown of life that God has promised to those who love Him.' The crown is given to the one who endures, not only to the one who wins.

Joni Erickson Tada and her friend Steve Estes have written a most insightful book about suffering; *When God Weeps*. Joni, in my opinion, is one of the most qualified people to write such a book. As a fit and healthy teenager, full of life and pulsating with energy, she had many plans for her future. However, on a balmy evening in Chesapeake Bay, as the sun began to set, she took a dive which was to change her life forever.

Nothing alerted her to the shallowness of the murky waters below her. Suddenly, she felt her head hit something unyielding and hard. There wasn't any pain. Just the sensation of a loud electrical buzz, and the sickening sound of crunching sand. Helplessly she lay among the stones and broken shells, held captive in a watery grave. Paralysis seized her, panic overwhelmed her and the possibility of death terrified her. Rescued only seconds before drowning by her sister Kathy, she was rushed by ambulance to the hospital. Surely, the numbness would wear off eventually. It never did! She sustained a diagonal fracture between her fourth and fifth cervical vertebrae, and that day became a quadriplegic. For the last fifty years, she has lived in a wheelchair with a broken neck and broken dreams. But not a broken spirit!

I think Joni has earned the right to ask the probing question "Is all the bleeding worth the benefit?" She answers by saying it's a matter of faith. It is like imagining a pair of scales; your pain on one side, and the glory your suffering is producing on the other side. Faith causes us to be like Rumpelstiltskin (in the fairy tale), weaving straw into gold. Just like a divine spinning wheel, our afflictions are producing for us an eternal weight of glory that will last forever.

J.B Phillips puts pain in perspective; 'The outward man does indeed suffer wear and tear, but every day the inward man receives fresh strength. These little troubles (which are really so transitory) are winning for us a permanent, glorious and solid reward out of all proportion to our pain.' (2 Corinthians 4:17 PHILLIPS). I love the way in which *The Message* expresses this same verse; 'Even though on the outside it often looks like things are falling apart on us, on the inside, where God is making new life, not a day goes by without His unfolding grace. These hard times are small potatoes compared to the good times, the lavish celebration prepared for us.'

When we finally step into the heavenly arena one day, we will see those who have been ravaged by pain, completely restored. My mum used to thrill at the thought of people she knew, now being in heaven. With a glint in her eye she would say to me, "Heather, we will all be perfect one day." But we're not in heaven yet!

Meanwhile, God doesn't simply leave us waiting with our noses pressed up against heaven's window pane. His wonderful work of healing starts now, while we're here on earth!

A crown of beauty *instead of* ashes.

The oil of joy *instead of* mourning.

A garment of praise *instead of* a spirit of despair.

A double portion *instead of* our shame.

An inheritance *instead of* our disgrace.

Plus…everlasting joy! (see Isaiah 61:3 and 7).

Now that's a great exchange rate right there!

So, in light of all this, my answer to the question "Will all the bleeding be worth the benefit?" has to be a resounding *Yes! Yes! Yes!* The Carpenters chisel will have done its work. The testing and the trials will be over. Then we'll hear those thrilling words, "Well done, good and faithful servant" (Matthew 25:23). On that day, every tear will be wiped away. All sighing will be gone. We'll bow before Him in adoration when we see His nail-pierced hands. Our own scars, the sorrows and sadness, the pain and anguish, will all fade away on that wonderful day. We'll look back and thank God He gave us the honor of suffering – for such a rich reward!

CHAPTER TWENTY-SIX

Pressed Grapes

The other day I was talking to Pastor Ray Andrews. (Someone who had previously received the benefit of Ray's wisdom, told me enthusiastically, "Everyone needs to see Ray!" Well sorry, they can't. He's too busy!)

However, he shared an interesting story with me. He had been counseling a multi-millionaire, who owned vineyards that spread across extensive hills and valleys. He explained that when the rains came they soaked the soil, but then gravity pulled the water further down the slopes, where the vine beds on the lower plains became submerged. There, the thirsty roots drank as much moisture as they needed for their fruits to become plump and ripe. Before long, they were ready for harvesting.

The grapes planted on the hillside however, did not enjoy such luxury. Their roots had to soak up whatever rains hung around long enough for them even to have a quick sip. Consequently, they didn't have the same opportunity to grow as plump and large as their more fortunate counterparts down in the valley. It wasn't fair, but what could they do? They were just grateful if they didn't end up looking like dried up prunes!

When the time came for the grapes to be gathered, the volume of the harvest in the valley was huge, unlike the yield from the hilly vines. (The disadvantaged fruits blushed red with embarrassment in comparison to their more favored friends!) After all the grapes had been picked, they were then pressed so the juice could be fermented and turned into wine. More bottles of wine were siphoned from the plump grapes, as one might expect. Not so many from the clusters on the hills.

Ray asked me, "Heather, how much do you think the wine cost that came from the valleys?" I had no idea. I appreciate a good wine, but I am certainly not a connoisseur! $30 a bottle was the correct answer.

"How much do you suppose the wine from the hilly country cost?" I thought it would be a lot less. How wrong I was. They sold each bottle for $300!

The illustration was clear. The grapes from the valleys looked delicious but were so saturated, they didn't taste nearly as sweet as the ones from the hills that had less water diluting their blood-red liquid. Initially, what seemed to be the more advantageous position for the vines to grow, was actually less beneficial in producing the more exquisite wines!

The analogy slipped perfectly into place. How similar in life. Not that this means God values one person more than another. He paid the same price for us all. However, it's clear that some people are a lot sweeter than others. Their painful experiences haven't left them sour and acidic with an astringent aftertaste in their lives, but have worked in them the rare vintage of trust.

Talk to the people who have suffered and who haven't had life easy. Listen to their Job-like stories. Savor the richness that pours from their hearts. Watch them as they yield graciously and walk with understanding. Admire the unconditional and sacrificial love they share. Notice how they quickly forgive and refuse to become bitter. Their lives have not been diluted with selfishness. Their words are flavored with kindness and their lives are seasoned with grace. They are not plump with self-importance. Life has been tough. They have been pressed and squeezed by their experiences. They haven't had the advantages that so many others have. However, like the vines on the hilly ground, the fruit from their lives has matured through their trials, and is delicious to taste.

Which bottle would you rather crack open with your à la carte meal? Which person would you rather be married to?

I know my answer!

Hannah's Story (1 Samuel 1-2)

Hannah is a woman in the Bible who is a great example our 'pressed grape' illustration. She was married to Elkanah. But, he was also married to a woman called Peninnah. (Understandably, there were going to be problems. Two wives! This never was going to be ideal!) Whether Hannah was the first or second wife we are not told, but Peninnah was her rival and leader of the opposition.

It was obvious that Hannah was her husband's favorite. He demonstrated his love by giving her double portions of food at the family sacrifices, which became the fertile soil for rampant jealousy! Peninnah despised Hannah, and expressions of hatred towards her knew no bounds.

However, there was a deeper agony that made matters worse. Hannah was barren and this hurt badly. The pain was like a searing burn that never seemed to heal. Peninnah scored highly because she was the mother of Elkanah's only sons and daughters. Every time one of the children ran past Hannah, the pangs of longing pierced her heart, reopening the gaping sore in her soul she so desperately tried to conceal.

It seemed that Peninnah was positioned in the 'valley' growing plump with children, while Hannah was stuck in the 'hilly' country, trying to produce fruit but could not. Admittedly, she was watered daily by her husband's loving affection, but the tormenting insults from 'the other wife' caused her joy to evaporate rapidly. Year after year, the merciless ridicule pierced her heart. Her infertility became a cloak of shame she wore for all to see. In those days, barrenness was considered a curse for any woman. But Hannah's name meant 'grace' (or 'favor'). Had God forgotten to be gracious to her? After all, children were believed to be a reward from the Lord. Then why was it that she couldn't give her husband children, while her rival popped them out like peas?

What makes the story even more poignant, is that we are told 'the Lord had closed her womb!' It wasn't her fault! She didn't know this though as she struggled to come to terms with her unfortunate lot. Her position and her condition caused her to become 'a woman of a sorrowful spirit' (or 'a woman who was deeply troubled').

She tried to disguise the shards of pain. Her husband knew, of course. It broke his heart, but what could he do? Wasn't the balm of his love enough to soothe away her sorrows? One day, he asked naively, "Am I not better to you than ten sons?" God bless him! At least he had great self-esteem!

One day, Hannah's heartache burst like a dam in her emotional river. (It wasn't a 'break-down' but a 'break-through' – to God!) Her pain gushed out and her tears overflowed in the temple of all places! All the family were celebrating at a feast, but Hannah had lost her appetite and didn't feel like eating. Unable to mask her anguish any longer, she left the table and went to pour out her heart to the Lord. She didn't make a scene. She didn't voice her bitterness. Only Eli the priest noticed her slumped down on the temple floor, as a pool of tears formed around her.

At that moment, Hannah attracted heaven's attention. (Tears always do!) Ushered in by her grief, she found herself in the throne room of God. Maybe she didn't know it. Maybe she didn't feel it. But that is where she was. Even so, Eli eyed her with suspicion. She mouthed some words but her voice made no sound. Surely, she was drunk! (I'm sure that many would have been driven to drink by this stage.) Not our beautiful Hannah.

"I was pouring out my soul to the Lord," she sobbed. "I have been praying here out of my great anguish and grief." Quickly, Eli realized his terrible mistake and changed his attitude. He never did discover what her problem was. (He didn't ask, and she didn't tell him!) But he knew God answered prayer. "Go in peace and may the God of Israel grant you what you have asked of Him."

At that moment, a divine river of peace began to surge through her soul. God had heard the cry of her heart! She went back and joined in the feast. She wasn't sad anymore. Her eyes may still have been red, but the sparkle in them returned.

Did anything outwardly change for Hannah? NO! She was still positioned up in the hilly country, but when the fruit of her life was harvested that year, it was the sweetest wine you ever tasted. God remembered her. He didn't forget her cries in the temple that day. Hannah conceived and gave birth to a son. She named him Samuel, saying, "Because I asked the Lord for him."

Not only did the wine pour forth in joyful gratitude, but it also contained the distinctive timbre of willing sacrifice. In our previous illustration, the grapes from the valley were plump and full of their own importance. Not this grape. The fruit of her life was dedicated to the Lord. Her prayer had not been about her looking good and competing with her rival. Her joy was not solely wrapped up in her baby, but in the Lord who had graciously removed her shame.

Fruit is best when it's ripe. Hannah's heart was ready. God had blessed her so richly that she wanted to give a gift herself. Faithfully she weaned her precious boy and prepared to offer him back to the Lord. "I prayed for this child, and the Lord has granted me what I asked of Him. So now I give Him back to the Lord. For his whole life, he will be given over to the Him." Words alone cannot convey the cost of this sacrifice. Her little son was the greatest treasure she had ever parted with, but she had no intention of taking him back. She was honored to relinquish the apple of her eye!

Here's the premium wine being poured out. The value is in the extravagance of love. Hannah isn't grasping and grabbing, holding the gift to herself. As a result, Samuel would eventually become one of Israel's greatest prophets. (Giving always yields a harvest!) What precious fruit!

Taste the sweetness of the wine that overflowed from her lips: "My heart rejoices in the Lord! Oh, how the Lord has blessed me! …No one is holy like the Lord! There is no one besides you; there is no Rock like our God"(1Sameul 2:1-2 NLT).

Here's the contrast between the fruit of the grapes: "She who was barren has borne seven children, but she who has had many sons pines way." Hannah's heart couldn't contain her gratitude to the Lord for delivering her from such disgrace and blessing her so richly; "The Lord sends poverty and wealth; He humbles and He exalts. He raises the poor from the dust and lifts the needy from the ash heap; He seats them with princes and has them inherit a throne of honor" (1 Samuel 2:5,7-8).

Perhaps we may wonder why Hannah had to go through such anguish of soul. Why did the Lord close her womb, allowing her to feel such shame? An illustration my daughter (also called Hannah) shared with me, may help us understand why we have to go through our own trials and suffering. She is a nursing educator, and told me about 'The First Pass Effect!' Maybe you, like me, have never heard of such a thing.

Some drugs, she explained, are administered orally, and some are given intravenously. The oral drugs are absorbed by the stomach and small intestine (gastrointestinal system) and transported to the liver, which filters out the poisons, protecting our bodies from any destructive toxins. When the drugs reach the liver, they metabolize. Chemical changes then take place to break down the medications, so they can be released back into the bloodstream and sent to where they are needed in the body.

The intravenous drugs do not have to be broken down and go through this process. I asked Hannah, "Why can't all drugs be given intravenously? It would be a lot quicker and save the liver so much work." (I am not a nurse, as you can tell!) Apparently, it is not only how rapidly the drugs will work, but it's also the most effective and safest way they are administered that is important. Some medicines, if given intravenously, would destroy the veins and could possibly be life-threatening.

How true to life! Some people just cruise along 'intravenously' without having to go through any major metabolic dramas. Yet the Lord in His wisdom may allow others to go through extreme trials in order for change to take place.

God closed Hannah's womb for His good and perfect reasons. In His time, and in response to her grief which she had poured out through prayer, He opened that same womb to bear the richest and rarest of treasures. The wine from her life was not acidic. Tears had tenderized her. Sorrows had softened her. Barrenness had broken her. Nevertheless, the 'metabolic' transformation was complete.

That is where the value of the pressed grapes comes from. Rare and expensive because of the multi-leveled taste, even though tears are often the moisture that help produce the full flavor. The fruit from Hannah's life changed a nation. Her son was powerfully used; divinely appointed to influence kings and anointed to speak God's Word to Israel. What a process to produce such an exquisite wine! Handpicked by the Lord and sovereignly harvested.

Psalm 126:5-6 says, 'Those who plant in tears will harvest with shouts of joy. They weep as they go to plant their seed but they sing as they return with their harvest" (NLT). In *The Message* we read, 'So those who planted their crops in despair…those who went off with heavy hearts will come home laughing, with armloads of blessing.' What a promise!

Our sowing may well be in sorrow, but our reaping will be with rejoicing. May the Lord help us to see that the seed of our sufferings will also yield a great harvest – the fruit of His Spirit in our lives!

'Pressed'　　　　　　　　H. Magee. 2016

Pressed to the point where all hope has gone,
Pressed, when the length of the trial is too long.
Pressed, so the crushing is too hard to bear,
Pressed, yet the wine is so rich and so rare.

Pressed beyond measure till your heart is breaking,
Pressed-grapes under pressure, for wine that God's making.
Pressed until there are no tears left to weep,
God's growing a harvest of joy we will reap!

(More Wine from the Grape Vine: A Message from Matt)

"If I believe the character of God and who He says He is, then I am able to trust Him. This brings up an interesting and challenging thought. I have seen both my parent's hearts break over me because of my illness. This has been so difficult to watch! If they were able to click their fingers and fix me in an instant, they would. The fact that they are unable, is simple. They are not God. If *they* love me as much as they do and *their* hearts break to the degree that they do, how much more so does God's heart? Yet He is able to heal me as quickly as the clicking of the fingers.

This is where trust begins. It is at this moment that believing God's Word becomes an action and not just a theoretical concept. If my parents could heal me, they would. God can heal, but as yet I am not healed. However, if I believe the reality of who God is, then I have to trust that something greater and deeper is happening on a spiritual level that I am unable to see or comprehend.

If my mother was able to heal me, but she also knew that my illness would greatly benefit and impact my life beyond anything I could think or imagine, it would not stop her heart from breaking. Nevertheless, it would stop her from clicking the proverbial healing fingers, because she would be short-circuiting a richness, not on an earthly value, but one of a spiritual value. If we believe what the Bible says about God, then our trust and belief has to follow, no matter what the situation is. If God says that He works all things

213

together for good, I need to believe it. Not in an authoritarian way, but from a place of peace. To the degree of trust, is the degree of peace. This doesn't change the situation you are in, but it changes how you walk out of it.

If my all-perfect, all-merciful, all-gracious loving Heavenly Father is not doing something in my life that I feel desperately needs to change, there must be a reason that far exceeds not being granted that request. Trusting God in such situations is the ultimate spiritual walk, so when I'm presented with one, I want to know that I can believe and thank God in all my circumstances. Just as the apostle Paul learnt – to be content, no matter what, because something far greater is happening beneath a surface too deep to see through. One day it will be revealed. As the scripture says, we see through a glass 'dimly' (translated also as 'darkly'). If that is the case, then I can rest in the knowledge that although I can't see the whole picture, God can! If what God says about Himself is true, even if my situation seems contradictory, then that's when trust is most needed and fully realized. If God is good, then I will believe that!

(Matt wrote this whilst recovering from a seizure! At the time of writing, there is still no medical help to stop him having four long non-epileptic seizures a day. His situation could not be darker for him at the moment. He could not feel more like a 'Pressed Grape.' But, taste the richness of the wine!)

CHAPTER TWENTY-SEVEN

Your Name is "Beloved"

We pastor a smaller church now since Len's stroke, but we love it! God meets with us each time we gather together, and our hearts are greatly strengthened by being in His presence.

Rob and Michelle are part of our church family. I had coffee with them today. Michelle's eyes moistened and Rob welled up with tears as they shared part of their journey with me. Sometimes, we have no idea the extremities people go through. How often pain is hidden behind gracious smiles and gentle eyes.

Michelle's walking stick and the difficulty she has in lifting her feet give part of her story away. She helped fill in some of the gaps in my understanding. Her father passed down a gene through the family that would cause all her sisters to suffer from of muscular dystrophy. Because the disease was hereditary, Michelle lived with the acute awareness of what she might eventually have to endure. The sinister symptoms remained dormant for over twenty years but eventually the silent darkness of her apprehension gave way to the dawn of reality .

As her symptoms became apparent, her legs began to feel like lead weights. Just walking a few steps felt as if she was dragging a ball and chain. Her hands started to lose their skillful dexterity. Her normal swallow reflex eventually slackened. Artificial tendons were attached to her drooping eyelids to prevent them constantly closing. Even breathing became labored and awkward.

"You know what I miss, Heather?" Her eyes glistened. "I miss dancing so much. I would go to the ballet and long for that feeling of freedom, more than words can say." It wasn't difficult to imagine her slight frame gliding gracefully through the air and pirouetting with ease However, those moments are now relegated to treasured memories. Just walking is awkward, let alone dancing.

"I used to love wandering through the shops, losing myself in retail therapy and the fun of trying on dresses, just because I could. I'd just hop in my car and go, when and wherever I wanted to. Now it has to be a 'one-stop-shop' and that's it!" Her visage darkened as if a cloud temporarily passed across her face. "I really regret the loss of my independence. These days I have to go with Rob and he hates shopping!" (Most men do, don't they? Go in, grab what they need because they know what they want, and then get out as quickly as possible. Not the best retail therapy companions!) Her countenance softened again, as though the sunlight had returned to brighten her gaze. Rob smiled with a knowing look as she teased him. "I have had to learn lots of patience through all this!" Now it was my turn to smile! I knew the Bible says that patience (or perseverance) is a mark of spiritual maturity (see Romans 5:3).

Isn't that why we are encouraged so often to wait *on* the Lord and wait *for* the Lord, and then just wait some more! Endurance and long-suffering are part of the fruit of the Holy Spirit that God is producing in our lives. Moment by moment and day by day, God is bringing us into situations that cause us to be dependent on Him.

Michelle agreed with her husband. "I've had to learn to rely on Rob so much more. That's been hard, because I have always been such an independent person." The sparkle in her eyes momentarily disappeared, obscured by a well of tears, but it soon resurfaced. (Joy searches like sunrays, to break through the clouds once again.)

"This experience has taught me so much. I'm really not bitter! It would have been easy to blame dad for this hereditary condition and even easier to blame God, but through it all, I've learned to rely on the Lord's strength. He has been so good to me. My family have also been amazing. Their unconditional love and support have been incredible, and the medical team who care for me have been so kind and understanding. I'm so grateful for all my many blessings!"

Blessings? Evidently, I was sitting in the presence of a rare and exquisite mature wine! Over the years, the sorrows in Michelle's life had ripened into a heartfelt appreciation of God's work in her life. He had allowed many trials to shape His image in her. She couldn't see what I saw. She was shining like a star against the dark backdrop of her disabilities.

Rob shone too, even though clouds had obscured his horizon some years ago, when he was diagnosed with Parkinson's disease. This physically debilitating condition can affect the sufferer in many ways, but the side-effects of the medications can be just as awful to endure. Rob certainly thought so. As we spoke, the strength in his voice weakened, a sign that our session should end soon. But not before a glint appeared in his eyes as they welled up with tears.

"You know, Heather, I was an alcoholic. It was nothing for me to spend $200 a week on liquor. It was getting me bad. I am also an asthmatic and have been found clinically dead on two occasions. My bronchial tubes all closed up on me, leaving me unconscious until medical help arrived on the scene. I wasn't even a Christian at that time, yet I found myself praying in the ambulance. If I had died then, I would never have had the privilege of knowing God's love as I do today. I am so very grateful!"

A few more tears fell down his cheeks, as the rich wine filtered through his heart. "God saved my life and this suffering we're going through now will all be over one day. In heaven, we will have brand new bodies. What hope we have. What amazing grace!

Our hearts had warmed with love as we'd spoken about God's goodness. Those who've suffered generally understand each other, even when their experiences are very different. Pain and sorrow are common denominators and magnetically draw people together who may never have felt that bond otherwise.

Eventually, it was time for us to go. Rob and I helped Michelle to her feet as they prepared to leave. I was deeply moved by their honesty and tender hearts. I knew life hadn't been easy for either of them. What they had shared with me had only taken two hours and was only the tip of the iceberg, yet the suffering they'd endured had lasted many years. But the fruit of their lives was mature and sweet. I could taste it!

One Sunday, when we were at church, Rob shared a prophetic message, which he felt God had laid on his heart. The frailty of his voice didn't lessen its impact. 'The Lord says, "Are you the one who I compelled to go through the hard places where I shaped you? Are you the one I walked with through the valley of tears, where I honed and tempered you? Are you the person you thought you would be? Are you the person you wanted to be? No, but you are the person I knew you would be, and I know your name...

...Your name is *Beloved!*"

What sweet wine poured over us that morning, and we drank it thirstily. People who haven't suffered don't appreciate comfort like those who have. The nature of comfort is to strengthen, soothe and encourage. People in pain thirst for the therapeutic wine of love and the relief of hope. God's love really is 'sweeter than wine' (Song of Solomon 1:2 NLT), and we are His beloved!

It just may be that the trials you are going through are the very means that the Lord is using to demonstrate His immeasurable love. David writes in Psalm 119:71-72, 'It was good for me to be afflicted that I may learn Your decrees. The law from Your mouth is more precious to me than thousands of pieces of silver and gold.' The paraphrase in *The Message* reads, 'My troubles turned out all for the best – they forced me to learn from your textbook. Truth from your mouth means more to me than striking it rich in a gold mine.'

Through their afflictions, Rob and Michelle have experienced God's grace and faithfulness in ways they would never have known otherwise. God is *good*. He knows what is *good* for us. Even our trials! He knows which ones are valuable and necessary in our lives.

And what we learn from them is more precious than gold!

CHAPTER TWENTY-EIGHT

Brokenness: The Wounding's of Divine Love

Have you ever been surprised when God has shown you what is really in your heart? Times of prolonged sickness can bring this revelation for sure! When our natural ability to bounce back has gone and our 'joie de vivre' evaporates, it is not always a pretty sight! So much of what we put our trust in has the ability to camouflage our vulnerability. Money will help to create pleasure for a season. Health can give us a false sense of well-being. Power may give us a sense of control. Any of these have the potential to feed our self-sufficiency, so we don't feel the need of God in our lives.

In the previous chapter, Michelle shared how she used to be such an independent person. If the truth is told, all of us are born with an inherent desire for freedom and independence from God.

We want to do everything in our own way and in our own time. We are all intrinsically selfish. The need for love and appreciation, the fight for survival and the desire for protection is instinctive. It can also be very strong. Some personalities are able to hide this better than others, but it's there all the same. At times these conflicts are intense.

God's colorful canvas of nature is a wonderful depiction of such struggles. The baby bee is a fascinating illustration. It starts off life as an egg in a six-sided cell. Three days later, it hatches into a small larva, whose goal in life is to eat as much as it can! Its growth is phenomenal during this stage, so to facilitate its growing body, it will shed its skin five times before hatching. Then, after a few days, worker bees seal the capsule with a porous capping of beeswax. In this secret place of hibernation, many changes take place; the eyes, legs and wings take shape. When the little larva has exhausted its supply of nourishment, it wraps itself tightly in a fine silk cocoon until the metamorphosis is complete. In due course, the young adult bee chews its way through the wax seal and finally breaks out of its confinement. As it emerges, the membrane encasing its wings rubs off. It is hard work and takes time. Nevertheless, in the difficulty of wrestling and wriggling, its wings are strengthened. Now it can fly. It's free at last!

Isn't that what happens to us? Life can be a struggle. Oh, but when we gave our lives to God, shouldn't that have been the end of all our problems? Weren't we meant to live happily ever after?

Wasn't this the beginning of a trouble-free zone, where God would answer our prayers in miraculous ways? Apparently not!

Jesus used an illustration from nature. In John 12:24 we read, 'Unless a kernel of wheat falls to the ground and dies, it remains only a single seed. But if it dies, it produces many seeds.' Inside that little grain of wheat, there is a germ of life. However, the external husk has to break open before the seed can germinate and grow. Through the invisible interaction of temperature and humidity, in that lonely, dark place under the ground, the outer protective casing is softened. The shell around the seed then splits open, and new life springs forth!

These are graphic pictures of what the Holy Spirit is doing in us. When we give our lives to Christ, His work of transforming us begins. It's like marriage really! Isn't falling in love the most exciting time in your life? The sense of being chosen and cherished. That's how it is when we become a Christian. God woos us and draws us by His love, finding a response in our hearts and a new relationship begins. He cares for us, comforts and encourages us. It's incredible! However, as with marriage, the ring goes on; then the real changes begin to take place! (Didn't anyone warn you?)

Wouldn't it be great if marriage was a continual extension of the honeymoon? No pressures; no in-laws (definitely), no members of the extended family around (hopefully), no household chores (delightfully), and no business commitments (absolutely). Just time to be together and enjoy some relaxed, stress-free days!

It certainly was for us. One evening, Len and I sat together on a huge rock at Land's End (in Cornwall, South of England), with our arms entwined around each other. Lost in our love, we gazed out to sea, captivated by the deep mango-yellow sunset, blissfully unaware of anyone or anything else. It's one of those special Kodak memories imprinted in my heart. If only that moment could have lasted forever!

Then we came home and it wasn't long before we had our first argument. (He was wrong, he must have been! It surely wasn't *my* fault!) What had I done to upset him so much? I was wide-eyed and innocent, and also quite naive. Moi? Didn't he love me anymore? Of course, he did. Just clash of wills, that's all. We were in the early stages of learning the wisdom of yielding!

It can be quite unnerving to see yourself in the true light of day. Compared to the romantic ambiance of the softly lit restaurants you visited during your heady courtship days, marriage is a place of broad daylight reality. However, in the safe atmosphere of trust and understanding, where the promise of cherishing hasn't faded, we then learn to adapt and blend together with the one we love.

We may well have to change, a lot! Sometimes we may struggle, like the bee bursting through the wax seal, or the tiny seed emerging from its shell. God may allow some dark and difficult situations for us to go through. Nevertheless, this is all part of the divine process of softening our hearts by His love so that His life can be released through us.

I remember reading about someone who had been working with elephants in Rangoon. They noticed there were willing workers and then there were 'sulkers.' There were those with gentle tempers and others who were angry and obstinate. The contrast was striking. Some elephants would drag a log that weighed two tons without a groan, while others, equally as powerful, were less willing and would make a fuss over a stick that weighed next to nothing.

We all have different strengths and weakness. Our characters and personalities are unique to each of us. Some yield more easily than others. But God knows the challenges that will change us. It's often though in these times that God steps in, shining the spotlight of His love upon us and begins to heal our broken hearts.

It happened to Peter, one of Jesus disciples. He didn't have any idea what was lurking deep inside his heart and what actions he was capable of. Was it possible that he would deny his best friend? Before Jesus went to the cross, He predicted His disciples would desert Him, but Peter was adamant. No way did that include him! "Even if all fall away on account of You, I never will." Jesus knew Peter better than Peter knew himself. Before the cock crowed twice that day, he would deny Him three times. And so he did!

In the soft firelight of a nearby courtyard, a humble servant girl recognized Peter as being one of Jesus friends. Then others levelled similar accusations at him. In the unbelievable pressure of an unpredictable moment, Peter spewed forth the most vehement profanities, denying he ever knew his Lord. His allegiance to Jesus just melted like wax in the heat of burning coals. Straight away, after those devastating words of denial, he remembered the prophecy about the rooster! Jesus had warned him. If only he had listened.

In that awful moment, Jesus turned around purposefully and looked directly at him. Peter's eyes met the gaze of God. Suddenly, the gravity of what he had done hit him. How could he have done this? He had let loose some serious emotions that day. In fact, he was so devastated by his brutal outburst, he broke down and wept. The shame and disgust that he had hurt his friend so much, crushed him more than words could say. His toughened kernel had cracked! This was one of the most defining moments in his life. Grace was about to do its perfect work.

Brokenness is the beginning of change, when our hearts begin to soften. God doesn't abandon us because we are broken. King David knew this first hand After he had sinned so greatly, he was devastated. Humbled and deeply sorry for all his failures, he wrote, "The sacrifice You want is a broken spirit. A broken and repentant heart, O God, You will not despise" (Psalm 51:17NLT). A broken spirit ushers us right into the courts of heaven. Pride slams the door! Spurgeon made the observation, 'This same experience is common to all the redeemed family of God, according to the degree in which the Holy Spirit has removed the natural heart of stone.' (A spiritual heart transplant!)

I remember when a dear friend rang us one day. He had been incarcerated for crimes committed many years before God saved

226

him. Many Saturday mornings he would ring from prison. On this particular day he said to me, "Heather, I am going to say something that you may think is strange. My time in jail has actually become a blessing to me! I am not the same any more. God has changed me! The garbage of my past has gone. I've been a great sinner, but I have been forgiven so much!" He then began to weep as the impact of his words resonated in his heart. "I am totally overwhelmed by God's love to me."

Here was a toughened man in prison, shedding tears out of his brokenness. Gone was his heart of stone. God had replaced it with a heart of flesh, softened by His love and forgiveness. Oh the value of tears, when we come to the end of ourselves and fall into the arms of the Lord. Here we find such loving acceptance and are filled with gratitude because God did not turn us away.

Peter was a completely different man from that day forward. New life burst forth and a new love overflowed that was visible for all to see. His passion was contagious. On the Day of Pentecost, he preached the greatest sermon of his life, all about his best friend. Such was the dynamic impact, that 3,000 people were converted. What a dramatic change! No longer was he ashamed, neither was he afraid. From being someone who denied even knowing Jesus, he became a man so filled with the power of the Holy Spirit, that he spoke about His Savior to thousands of people. (See Acts 2)

Later, Peter wrote to reassure God's people in their trials; 'In this you greatly rejoice, though now for a little while you may have had to suffer grief in all kinds of trials. These have come so that your faith–of greater worth than gold, which perishes even though refined by fire–may be proved genuine and may result in praise, glory and honor when Jesus Christ is revealed' (1 Peter 1:6-7).

Perhaps we may wonder why it is necessary for God to test the genuineness of our faith. 'Genuine' means real and authentic. Can some faith be fake? Sometimes! Only recently, I saw how vitally important it is to know the difference. My friend Paul and I were photographing some spectacular looking diamonds in the back of a jeweler's shop. (One of those photos is now on the back cover of this book!) We had set up the lights, hand-picked the jewels and carefully arranged them on a dark gravel backdrop, to display their beauty and capture their brilliance.

We hadn't been there long, when we were distracted by a loud, animated conversation taking place in the front of the shop. A couple of women were trying to sell some pieces of platinum. (This was also a pawnshop, where the jeweler bought and sold rare treasures.) One of them produced her ID and proceeded to state her exorbitant price. Unbeknown to her, the owner of the shop had received a disturbing call earlier in the day. It was from another jeweler in the same locality, warning he had just been ripped him off by people selling him forged platinum for thousands of dollars! Now here they were trying to scam our friend, right before our eyes!

With absolute professionalism, he asked to see the hallmark that would verify the platinum's authenticity. As though nothing was even remotely suspicious, he continued his questioning. At the same time, a call was made to the police, alerting them of a possible crime being played out blatantly before us. Because the jeweler is so experienced at discerning what is and is not real, he picked the fraud immediately. Soon the culprits were in the capable hands of the law. These women were asking thousands of dollars for something that was not genuine. What they presented as pure platinum was only cleverly disguised raw metal! Clever, but not smart!

How important to know what is authentic! How even more necessary to know what is fake, because both can appear exactly the same. One is genuine and highly valuable; the other is counterfeit and consequently worthless. Pressure reveals what is authentic, and so does heat. Will we melt in the fire? Will we buckle, and crumble in a heap? Is our faith genuine? We'll soon know!

Peter's love for Jesus was tested. He had buckled for sure! He knew that he had hurt Jesus deeply. Would he eventually receive the stinging rebuke he justifiably expected? Thankfully not! Peter had chastised himself enough. He'd wept a river already. Jesus was eager to restore their relationship.

After a meal together, around another coal fire, Jesus drew his friend aside. There was something he wanted to know. Poignantly, He asked, "Do you love me?" This was a cutting moment. Peter knew precisely what Jesus was referring to; those dreadful denials that had understandably caused Jesus to doubt his love. If only he had stood with Jesus in His hour of trial. If only he could turn back the clock. But he couldn't!

However, Peter remembered when he had been with Jesus and a sinful woman had poured an expensive alabaster box of perfume over His head. "She was forgiven many, many sins, and so she is very, very grateful" (Luke 7:47 *The Message*). Peter was very thankful too! "Yes Lord, You know that I love You!" He genuinely did. He could easily have run away, driven by the shame of his failures. But he didn't! He was so grateful to have been forgiven. So glad not to get what he so rightly deserved. (Aren't we all!)

No further questions were asked. There was no chastisement or harsh rebuke. No silent treatment. In fact, that was the moment when Jesus reinstated Peter and recommissioned him. "Feed my lambs and take care of my sheep…Follow me." Peter didn't have to think twice. Unconditional love is irresistible!

A tale of two doggies

One day, I was walking back home from the park with my dog Mollie. As I reached my driveway, there stood the most gorgeous puppy, looking quite lost. She didn't have a collar with any ID, so finding her owner was not going to be easy. She just looked at me plaintively and jumped up as far as her legs would reach, pleading to be held.

Instantly, I fell in love with this little pooch. Her coat was a soft ginger color. I imagined Mollie and my new nameless friend quickly learning to like each other. (Sadly, a rare virus had recently taken our other beautiful doggy Mishka, so I knew I could make room for one more!) However, I should at least try to find its owner first before I became too enthusiastic. I didn't recognize it as being a local puppy. We know and love all the dogs in the neighborhood (well, most of them), so who belonged to this one? Surely, someone would be missing her by now.

Our neighbor Joe suggested that the puppy might have come from a house just along the street as he had seen it hanging around there earlier in the day. My daughter Hannah offered to investigate, and it wasn't long before she returned with a woman walking briskly beside her.

"Thank-you so much." Her words tumbled out in gratitude. "I was doggy-sitting for my daughter. I'd only just noticed the puppy had disappeared. She is so naughty, (referring to the dog!) Give her half a chance and she's gone. Today, I left her playing in the back yard and while I was at work, she's dug her way out under the fence. I didn't know where to find her!"

Funnily enough, I couldn't imagine Mollie trying to run away. We leave the gate open when we garden or take the garbage out and she just sits there patiently until we come back in. Then she wags her tail, welcoming us again as though we had been away for hours! There's nothing in her that wants to leave. Why would she? She is unconditionally loved, highly treasured…and very well fed. She's one discerning doggy!

231

Why would anyone want to walk away from God? Do we treat our animals better than God cares for us? But many people stopped following Jesus, even after the life-changing miracles He had done for them. One day, He asked His disciples, "You do not want to leave too, do you?" It was Peter who replied, "Lord, to whom shall we go? You have the words of eternal life. We believe and know You are the Holy One of God" (John 6:67-68). He spoke for them all. Jesus had revolutionized their lives. Where *would* they go in search of such love? Why *would* they want to go anywhere else?

Our son Matt has written a song called 'Distant Sands.' Inside the CD cover he writes, "God loves us so much. How can we begin to express this? 'We love Him because He first loved us.' He stands on the shoreline of our lives and draws us to Himself."

Distant Sands

A broken vessel washed on the sands

You mend, restore, with outstretched hands.

This life within Your Son I must

Lay me down, in You I trust.

Was torn and broken in my sin.

You clothed me, gave me shelter, took me in.

And on that day before the dawn

My heart was healed, no longer torn.

This could almost have been written for Peter. Perhaps for us also?

CHAPTER TWENTY-NINE

The Key to Contentment

When there are times we're left breathless with bewilderment, it's encouraging to listen to others who have suffered, and plumbed deeper depths than we have, because they've experienced, and consequently understand what they are talking about.

I mentioned Joni Eareckson in a previous chapter. Living fifty years as a quadriplegic, Joni has surely earned enough battle stripes to warrant giving us her definition of suffering. It sounds so simple and yet it's profound; She says, "Suffering is having what you don't want and wanting what you don't have!" How true!

Joni explained that after her diving accident, she felt trapped and totally helpless, imprisoned in her own body. Her confinement compelled her to look at someone else who had been held captive;

the apostle Paul. He knew what it was to be under house arrest and constantly watched by guards. He had been thrown into a few dark and dingy prison cells, just for sharing the Good News about God! His feet had been fettered, and his back whipped like a plowed field. He had been stoned and left for dead. He knew what it was to suffer in ways that most of us never will. (Hopefully!)

Nevertheless, Paul had learned to be content 'whatever.' He was able to say, "I know what it is to be in need, and I know what it is to have plenty. I have learned the secret of being content in any and every situation, whether well-fed or hungry, whether living in plenty or in want" (Philippians 4:12). As a result, even when he was locked up behind bars, Paul could say, "Rejoice in the Lord always!" What a heart at peace with God. Contentment and joy go together.

One time, Paul was imprisoned with his friend Silas (Acts 16). They had been preaching and were on their way to a prayer meeting, when suddenly they were dragged into the market place, beaten, and incarcerated within four cold stone walls! With their feet in shackles and their wrists in chains, they were impounded behind the guarded doors of a dark dungeon. But, God wasn't locked out of their cell. He was there with them, throughout their whole ordeal.

The flame of God's love was unquenchable. Hadn't they been on their way to pray? What was stopping them now? Prison doors couldn't bar their way to an audience with the King of Heaven! Softly spoken prayers began to bubble up and cascade into songs of praise, as though they had a whole choir within them. Together they sang into the heavens. The other prisoners listened, astonished at the rapturous melodies infiltrating their adjoining cells. Honored to be persecuted for God's name, their hearts overflowed with joy.

Then, at midnight it happened! They shook, but not with fear. A powerful earthquake rumbled beneath them, increasing with such force that the floors began to dance. The doors sprung open. Their chains fell loose, unlocked by an invisible hand. Paul and Silas were released, all because of a worship service at midnight. They weren't singing because escape was at hand. They didn't have one eye on the window and one eye on the Lord. They were content to have both eyes on God and leave their predicament with Him. And look what happened!

From her observations of decades in a wheelchair, Joni says, "When life isn't the way you like it, like it the way it is…one day at a time with Christ. And you will be blessed" This opens the flood gates to God's peace joy and rest, that money could never buy. So many try to use health, beauty, power and possessions to fulfill their insatiable longings. How much wiser are we to adjust our desires to fit in with our circumstances.

Understanding this has helped me greatly. Did I ever suppose my life would turn out the way it has? Not for one minute! Did I expect that my husband would suffer a stroke at such a relatively young age? Did I think that my daughter would drown and be under water for almost nine minutes when she was only three years old?

(Or envisage seeing God's amazing miracle to our family, when she was brought her back to life, just moments from brain death!) Did I contemplate being diagnosed with Type 1 diabetes and twice with cancer? Never in my wildest dreams. Did I assume that I'd have to care so many years for my son and watch someone I love so much, suffer so greatly? No way in the world!

Nevertheless, it's just the way life has been and it's just the way life is. But, I'm learning to like it as it is, whether I like it or not! I'm learning to trust God knows what's best for me and that He has me in exactly the right place with the right people at the right time. I'm learning to be content. I did say 'learning!' I have a lot more to learn and so much more to understand. Yet, it has been amazing. I have experienced more joy than should naturally be possible. It's God's peace; His peace that passes all understanding.

I'm not alone, and neither are you if you know the Lord. His presence can turn your prison into a palace!

CHAPTER THIRTY

Some Will, Some Won't

Why will some people be healed and others won't? This is a difficult question. When I discovered I had cancer, Len and I prayed fervently that I would be healed. My friends prayed for me. Pastors prayed. Healing Evangelists laid their hands on me in faith. Yet I wasn't healed. I still had to go through the double mastectomy which I had been assured was God's path of life for me.

I continue to struggle with Type 1 diabetes, which requires me to test my blood sugars and inject myself with insulin about 5 times a day. Len prayed for one woman when he was speaking on a radio broadcast who had the same condition as I have and she was healed! So why wasn't I healed when Len and others prayed for me? This isn't an easy question, although I believe the best answer lies in the loving heart of God's purposes and sovereign will. Some of God's children are saved *from* walking through the fires of life. Some are saved *in* the fiery furnace. Both experiences have their place in our lives. In either situation, we will have a testimony to the faithfulness of God.

A few years ago, there were two men in our church who both had prostate cancer. One of them was miraculously healed and the other wasn't, even though he was prayed for by the same people. Why was this? Doesn't God always answer prayer the way we want Him to? Wasn't it His will that they were both healed, so their faith would be encouraged by experiencing God's power?

The one who did get healed wasn't a Christian at the time, so it certainly wasn't his great faith that brought about the miracle! He just wept with gratitude and gave his life to Jesus. Our friend often weeps. God saved his life in more ways than one! He's been totally overwhelmed in experiencing such grace.

Our other friend who didn't get healed was an older Christian and well established in his faith. You might have thought it would be the other way around; the one with greater faith would more likely be healed than the other who hardly had any at all. However, grace cannot incur a debt. Grace would not be grace if it could be earned in any way!

When we pray therefore, we must leave the results with God. He is sovereign and ultimately, it's His decision. He knows what is the best for us in every situation.

Paradise Lost

We live in a broken world. Listening to the stories of people's lives makes that very clear! We won't realize the enormity of what happened to us though, unless we understand the catastrophe that took place in the Garden of Eden, when sin entered into our world (Genesis 2-3). God never intended sickness and death to be part of His original creation.

When God created the heavens and the earth, He saw 'all that He had made, and it was very good!' He created man, and fashioned the most beautiful woman for him as his partner. Both were made in His image. He also gave them the most luxuriant garden to live in, filled with all kinds of trees, laden with fruit, with a magnificent river to water the land. (Sounds amazing. It was perfect!)

Except, there was a serpent creeping around behind the scene. He was coiled, ready for his entrance into the drama. Eventually, the moment presented itself. God had warned Adam, "You are free to eat from any tree in the garden; but you must not eat from the tree of the knowledge of good and evil, for when you eat of it you will surely die." The devil had been listening intently, waiting for his cue. Now was his time to act.

Slithering into the story, he hid in the shadows for Eve. Upon her arrival. he arced up and hissed, "Did God really say you must not eat from any tree in the garden?" Without missing a beat, she replied, "Yes, we can eat the fruit from all the trees, except one; the tree in the middle of the garden. We're not to eat its fruit and we're not even to touch it, or we will die." Both Adam and Eve clearly knew the deal.

"You don't actually believe that, do you?" the serpent quizzed mockingly. "Of course you won't die! Eat! Especially from the tree of the knowledge of good and evil. That's the best tree of all. Then your eyes will be opened. Spiritual enlightenment is what you need. Then you'll be like God!"

The thought was captivating. It sounded feasible. Eve salivated over the idea of tasting the delicious looking fruit. Perhaps it would give her special powers. Perhaps it would also make her a whole lot wiser. The serpent seemed to think so. Maybe he was right and God hadn't really meant what He'd said. So she talked herself right into succumbing to the deadliest temptation of all – ignoring God!

Unfortunately, the serpent was partly right in what he said. In eating the deadly fruit, their eyes were opened, but what they saw wasn't good. Suddenly they realized that they were naked. Now they knew goodness second hand and evil first hand. Shock and horror! Not a pretty sight. Quickly they grabbed some fig leaves and clothed themselves with the foliage.

When Adam and Eve ate the fruit that fateful day, something cataclysmic and eternally devastating happened. Rebellion found a home in man's heart. Disobedience sowed its rotten seed in the soil of man's soul. Now God couldn't trust them to fulfill the purpose for which they had been created. Instead of having a friendship with this first couple, He found them hiding fearfully amongst the trees.

God's questions pierced them like arrows. "Where are you? What have you done? Did you eat the fruit from that tree I told you not to?" What could they say? They understood what God had said to them, but they thought they knew better.

Smarting, Adam blamed his wife *and* God. "It was the woman *You* put here with me. *She* gave me some fruit from the tree!" Then indignantly, Eve accused the serpent. God nailed each one. Curses for all of them. Rebellion had given birth to sin. God's perfect world had been contaminated and permanently stained. Now they would all suffer the consequences of such an unbelievable violation against their Creator.

Adam and Eve were immediately ordered to leave the garden forever. Powerful cherubim were placed at the gate, guarding the entrance with a flaming sword that flashed incessantly. They would never come back! From the mountain heights of having the closest relationship with God, they plunged down into the deepest ravine, and brought the rest of the world abseiling with them. We all caught the sin virus that day and we all suffer because of it.

God knew this would happen, which is why He planned our salvation long before He ever made the world. That blows my mind. God was thinking about you and me before He ever made one tree or filled one ocean. Jesus came to take our punishment, so we might be saved. Our spirits have been 'redeemed,' meaning 'delivered by payment of a price' – as in slaves being set free. Jesus became the slave! His death was the price he paid so the guilty could go free!

However, unlike our spirits, *our bodies haven't been redeemed yet*. Paul says in Romans 8:22-23, 'We know that the whole creation has been groaning as in the pains of childbirth right up to the present time. Not only so, but we ourselves…groan inwardly as we wait eagerly for…'*the redemption of our bodies.*' Or, as the NLT states; 'We too, wait anxiously for the day when God will give us our full rights as His children, including *our new bodies He has promised us.*' (Emphasis mine.) We are indeed living in a 'fallen' world, but God hasn't left us without hope. There are times when He intervenes with merciful displays of love in our lives. Over the years, we have had the honor of witnessing some amazing miracles.

One of our friends had a condition called 'silent reflux' (when the valve controlling the acid in the stomach is not able to function properly). Kay had suffered burning in her esophagus for years, but the drugs that she had been taking to minimize the pain were no longer having any effect. Her distress was extreme; she could barely swallow. Sometimes so much acid would creep up her throat, that it felt as if she was having a heart attack! A hacking cough persisted night and day. She propped herself up in bed with four large pillows, as sleep was almost impossible for any significant length of time. Unfortunately, her last life-line of hope was a laparoscopic gastric band operation. Reluctantly she grasped it both hands, and so the date was scheduled.

Nevertheless, one week before the surgery, her husband gently persuaded her to ask for prayer at church. In her own words she told me, "Heather, I was so ill and miserable. I had never felt more unspiritual in my whole life! Because I had been working so hard at the time, I thought I had brought this on myself and that I was to blame for this awful situation. So I didn't even think to ask God for healing!' (Grace would not be grace if miracles were given in direct proportion to certain levels of faith. Thankfully, miracles are God's undeserved love-gifts.)

Kay needed a miracle and so gave in to her husband's coaxing. Len and I were overseas at the time, so one of the other leaders in our church took the meeting. He asked an elderly lady sitting at the back of our congregation to come and pray for her. Everyone else gathered around, joining their hearts with her in faith. Kay says that suddenly she felt a warm sensation, as if liquid honey was washing over her. Her husband noticed her face was literally glowing.

After the service, they both went out to have lunch together. Looking at his watch, her husband remarked that one full hour had passed and she hadn't coughed. She still hasn't! Kay was completely healed. The doctors were amazed! They knew how seriously ill she had been. The operation was canceled and her drugs were no longer needed, because God graciously answered an elderly lady's prayer! Incredibly, about one month later, the same dear lady who prayed for our friend, suddenly passed away herself. Len took her funeral! Some will get healed. Some won't. It's God's call!

Another of our friends had pancreatitis and was only given a 5% chance of survival. Len and I went to pray for her in the hospital as she lay there fighting for her life. I sat next to her on the side of the bed and came close to pulling out her drains accidently, which were hidden under the bedclothes! This could have been disastrous! Fortunately, it wasn't, so after we recovered from the shock of my mistake, we prayed for her and a few days later she was well enough to be discharged from hospital. Now, that's not to detract from the doctor's expertise and their excellent medical treatment. God works in many ways in answer to our prayers, but she knew her recovery was an absolute miracle.

On another occasion, we were called to the home of a friend of ours, whose 9-year-old son was dying of cancer. His mum and dad weren't Christians at the time. I remember the day well, because Len's pastor was visiting from England, so he joined us. (The more people praying at times like this always feels better!) We prayed up a storm. Even the neighbors must have wondered what the ruckus was all about think? It didn't matter. We were banging on Heaven's door, pleading with God for this little boy. My heart was breaking to see this mother's pain! We were desperately asking for a miracle.

After a couple of weeks, I felt an urgency to go and visit the family again. My sister Libby came with me. We found ourselves walking into a sea of sadness. Their precious boy was in a coma and fading fast. The other members of the family had gathered around to support each other, while waiting for his final moment. Gladly, they gave us their permission to pray for him. Libby and I tiptoed beside his bed. I wrapped my arms around his head and then began to call upon the Lord for their son. My heart is also a mother's heart. My children were a similar age at the time. This was deep anguish and excruciating agony.

I asked God to take this little one's life in His hands and save him. Before I had finished praying, Libby whispered nervously, "I think he's gone!" Her eyes were pinned on him all the way through our prayer. God answered at that very moment, releasing him from his struggle. He had been so brave and fought such a courageous fight. Finally, it was over. Now he was free.

The Sunday after her son's body was lowered into the ground, his heartbroken mother found solace in the 'God of all comfort.' Len gave an invitation at church for those who wanted to receive Jesus as their Savior. She knew her son was in heaven. She longed to see her son again, but she also realized that to see him, she must go where he had already gone. Jesus was the way, so she opened her heart to Him. A little seed had fallen into the ground, and it didn't remain alone (see John 12:24).

Here we see three very different scenarios. The Lord acted in each of these situations! He healed our friend with her serious reflux problem. He healed our other friend with pancreatitis. But He took the young boy to be with Him in heaven. All of them were answers to prayer, and each one was planned in the heart of God.

God does intervene at times and it's incredible when He does, albeit, we still live in a broken world. Disasters strike and accidents occur due to the natural laws of cause and effect. Heat makes ice melt, which may cause icebergs to drift and float into the sea paths of ocean liners like the Titanic. Did God make the Titanic sink? No, natural forces played their part. Sadly, tragedies do happen! It's just the way it is. Yet God remains just and sovereign at all times.

Understanding this helps me surrender my life into His hands and trust His decisions for my life. He will always answer my cries for help, in the way *He knows is best*, and in His perfect timing.

CHAPTER THIRTY-ONE

The "D" Word!

Death is not the most popular selection on the menu of life. We don't choose to sample its bitter spices, even though it will be served up to us all one day! Enoch and Elijah are the only ones referred to in the Bible who left this life without experiencing its unpalatable taste. (Their 'departures' were supernatural!) Except for those who are still living when Jesus returns, the rest of us will die one day. Those dates and occasions are recorded in heaven, for a time and place we aren't privy to for now.

It is going to happen, so I think it is worth talking about here. If you would rather not think about it yet, please feel free to turn the next few pages. However, God's Word has much to say about it, and we would be wise to prepare for its eventuality.

Death is the experience we must all go through to enter into eternity. It was said at one funeral, "Don't enter the box unless your exit is clear!" (Good advice!) It's imperative we know where we're going to spend our eternity. It's the doorway to heaven for all who have trusted in Jesus as their Savior and have been born into God's family. When God is your Father, heaven is your spiritual home.

I remember many times I shared with my mum about heaven. Death for her was not some dreadful event to be feared. In fact, in Psalm 116:15 we read, 'precious in the sight of the Lord is the death of His saints.' David says in his shepherd psalm, "Even though I walk through the valley of the shadow of death, I will fear no evil, for You are with me" (Psalm 23:4). God is going to be there with us, as He has been all our lives. This time though, we will 'put off' our natural bodies, as if we're taking off an old jacket and putting on our heavenly robes.

The apostle Paul says, "…We know that when these bodies of ours are taken down like tents and folded away, they will be replaced by resurrection bodies in heaven – God-made, not handmade – and we'll never have to relocate our "tents" again…Compared to what's coming, living conditions around here seem like a stopover in an unfurnished shack, and we're tired of it! We've been given a glimpse of the real thing, our true home, our resurrection bodies! The Spirit of God whets our appetite by giving us a taste of what's ahead. He puts a little of heaven in our hearts so that we'll never settle for less" (2 Corinthians 5;1-5 *The Message*).

When I read these verses, I can feel the longing in Paul's heart. There is no tinge of fear. In fact, he's admitting his preference to be at home with His Savior, who he has willingly served all his life. He knows that heaven is going to be so wonderful. In Revelation 21:4 (KJV) we read, 'There shall be no more death, neither sorrow, nor crying, neither shall there be any more pain: for the former things are passed away.' (Sounds like heaven to me!) A brand-new eternal day will dawn for each of us on our heavenly birthday. This fills us with expectation; it inspires us with motivation to run our race with joy and perseverance. We don't have to be fearful of its eventuality.

When Jesus told his disciples that He was going to be leaving them soon, they asked where He was going. They wanted to go with Him. That was when Jesus said to them, "Do not let your hearts be troubled. Trust in God, trust also in Me. In My Father's house are many rooms." This is the perfect advice for us when thinking about the time when we will follow the Lord to heaven. "Don't be afraid! I am going to prepare a place for you, and I will come back and take you to be with me, that you also may be where I am" (John 14:1-3). Heaven is our Father's house! We're going to live with Him forever. This is the glorious hope that fortifies us, when understandably, we may feel afraid. It won't be long! Life is short. Eternity is not!

The Bible uses many different analogies to describe the brevity of life. It says that our days pass as briefly as…'A breath, a vapor or a puff of smoke, a tale that is told, water spilled on the desert floor, one who wakes from sleep, a dream, a weaver's shuttle, a cloud that vanishes, a tent that is pitched.' Nothing stays the same. Everything is transient. We are just passing through life to our heavenly home as travelers and strangers. The more we get to know God, the more we will love Him, because we'll keep on discovering how wonderful He is. The more we love Him, the more we'll long to be with Him. And He loves us more than we can ever imagine!

God's Treasured Possessions

In Malachi 3:16-17 we read, 'Then those who feared the Lord talked with each other and the Lord listened and heard.' The Lord hears when we talk about Him. God loves it when what matters to Him, also matters to us. His heart is touched and thrilled whenever we mention His name. He even makes a record of it on heavenly parchment: 'A scroll of remembrance was written in His presence concerning those who feared the Lord and honored His name.'

"They shall be Mine," says the Lord of hosts,

"On the day that I make them My jewels" (NKJV).

The Hebrew word used here is 'segullah,' meaning 'special treasure' (as in the royal treasures belonging to a king). How awesome is this! Those who have been born into God's family by faith in Jesus, are going to be part of His treasure chest when He collects His jewels in eternity. "You will be a crown of splendor in the Lord's hand, a royal diadem in the hand of your God" (Isaiah 62:3).

However, we have not been placed in God's crown yet. God is still searching for His jewels and skillfully shaping each one. Each precious stone has its own inestimable value and beauty. When each one has been found, they will be washed and highly polished. Then with great joy, when the preparation has been done, when the trials and the tribulations have finished their work, the Lord will set us in His crown as a reflection of His glory.

In Isaiah 54:11-12 we also read, "Oh afflicted city, lashed by storms and not comforted. I will build you with stones of turquoise, your foundations with sapphires. I will make your battlements of rubies, your gates of sparkling jewels and all your walls of precious stones." If you feel that you are being pummeled by afflictions and lashed by storms, be encouraged. God hasn't forgotten you. Out of the pounding force of the tempest, God shapes and fashions us, so as to make us sparkle with His beauty and honor!

We are God's treasured possession. One day, He will take us to heaven and place us where we will display His glory best. For the Christian, death is when this will happen. Even our loved ones are only loaned to us as precious gifts along life's journey. They don't belong to us permanently. Eventually they must return to the One who so kindly lent them to us in the first place. It is God who takes them, in His perfect timing.

It just so happens I am going to the funeral of the dear woman whose husband hung himself above the altar of a Roman Catholic Cathedral! (I mentioned her in the introduction of this book.) She remarried and continued to raised her three boys, yet today we will celebrate the fact that the Lord has taken her home to be with Him.

She suffered greatly, but the waves that buffeted her during her life have done their work. Recently she rededicated her life to the Lord. Now she will shine as one of God's precious jewels and throughout eternity, she will reflect His wonderful grace in saving her forever.

Then I remember Annie. Dear sweet Annie. After her funeral, I wrote in my journal;

'Annie's triumphal entry into heaven! A time to be born, and a time to die; a time to plant, and a time to uproot (Ecclesiastes 3:2). Thank-you Lord, for delivering Annie from her body, racked with pain and suffering. How she has labored this last month, yet what a joy and inner sense of Your presence she has experienced. As her doctor said today, "Annie is a special lady; she has given much more to us than we ever gave to her." He was so right.

Three days ago, she told us she saw angels who came into her hospital room and stood at the end of her bed. She even described their distinctive features; "They were huge with beautiful smiling faces, dressed in golden robes. They didn't come through the door, they just appeared from over there." She pointed towards the wall directly opposite, where there was actually no opening at all. They had just come to be with Annie for a brief moment, reassuring her she was not alone. I'm sure they were waiting to escort her to glory!

Thank-you Lord for opening Annie's eyes to the realities of heaven! Now she's in Your presence, cocooned in Your love forever, I could not have wished for her to stay any longer, and she didn't want to either. She was ready to go Home. Now she's there in Your perfect timing; not one minute too soon and not one second too late.

Thank-you Lord for Annie's shining example of dying by faith. She was a great testimony, joking right up to our last conversation when she was almost too weak to laugh. She pleaded with Len to stop his jokes, as her sides hurt from laughing. I'm sure she'll have the greatest sense of humor in heaven. She'll be able to sing with the best set of lungs (she had lung cancer). She sang in our worship team, but eventually she couldn't sustain the melodies. Breathing became arduous and standing was exhausting. (Not anymore!)

Annie's life has touched so many people. May they know it was You Lord, who transformed the sufferings of her life and made her into such a trophy of grace. What a work of art from the Potter's hand. You took her as the hard lump of clay she was when You found her, and fashioned her into the beautiful vessel she became. We stood back amazed to see the transformation, as her tears turned to laughter and her sorrows to joy. So, thank-you Lord for Annie. May her courage always inspire me to praise and trust You, even when all natural hope fades away,

...for You remain faithful!'

~~

Sometimes we sing a song in church that was written by Chris Lambe. The lyrics were penned after a life-changing experience of intense suffering. Inside the cover of his CD he writes, 'A few years ago I was afflicted with cancer. Fortunately, by the grace of God, I am well now and have emerged from this whole incident a far better person. "Layer upon Layer" are inadequate words trying to express the great and marvelous work of God who, by His grace, in every circumstance, weaves His beautiful tapestry into our lives to bring about the character of Christ.' I love this song. It helps us see what God is doing in our lives, from His perspective.

Layer upon layer He touches so gently,
His hand comes to me like the dew on the morn,
So softly, so surely; patiently, purely
He fashions His child as the dawn.

Great are Your marvelous works, oh Lord
Bringing us into Your likeness.
Day after day through the trials and the storms
Your work continues in me.

See it unfolding the work of the Master
Day after day, till the new day has come,
So beautifully dawning, perfectly forming
Shining like gold in the sun.

Soon we'll be standing arrayed in His glory,
The work of His grace will be finally done.
So skillfully woven, wonderfully chosen,
Shining like gold in the sun.

Anthony Norris Groves, (considered by many to be the father of faith missions) said during the last week of his life, 'How precious it is to feel that all these human ills are, to the redeemed of the Lord, what the chariots of fire were to Elijah, alarming to look at but the Father's way of bringing his own Home.' He was not afraid. He had learned the benefit of bowing to God's sovereign will, knowing He lovingly appoints our daily measure of suffering. Therefore, he was able to say, 'Even so Father, for so it seemed good in Thy sight.'

How good is this! We are going 'Home!' But, we're not there yet. For now, we press on, running to reach the end of our race, '…for the prize of the high calling of God' (Philippians 3:14 KJV). We will never be able to express our absolute joy and amazement when we realize what the Lord has prepared for those who love Him. Death is just the doorway into the awesome reality of our eternal destiny.

By God's grace, I'll see you there!

CHAPTER THIRTY-TWO

Different Scenarios for Different Portfolios

The Lord doesn't always work exactly the same way in our lives. Sometimes, God may save us from having to fight a particular battle, and He will protect us from the attacks of our enemies (both physically and spiritually). At other times, however, God may allow us to engage in the battle, so we'll see His deliverance on our behalf.

Jehoshaphat, one of the kings of Judah in the Old Testament, is a great example of how God uses each of these different scenarios in our lives. During the early years of his reign he was spared many conflicts. He was a good king. When he was young he walked in the ways of his father, David. He didn't worship Baal. He honored God in the decisions he made for his nation. He was devoted to the Lord. Everyone knew that God was with him.

The surrounding nations knew too. They had heard how God was protecting His people in miraculous ways, so they were afraid to go to war against Jehoshaphat. In fact, it was quite the opposite; some of them even brought him presents! They gave him silver and flocks of rams and goats. Life was great for this new king. He was flanked by faithful men. He strengthened his position with fortified cities. He had money, power and prestige! If only things could have stayed just the way they were. They didn't! (see 2 Chronicles 20.)

Suddenly, out of the blue, a frantic knock on the door alerted King Jehoshaphat to the fact that he was in serious trouble! Some men with an urgent message fell before him. "It's not good news, O king. A vast army is marching against you and has congealed like a massive thunderhead. The storm clouds of war are gathering, and could burst at any moment!"

The Moabites and the Ammonites were indeed a 'vast army!' Now what was he going to do? He was alarmed. He wasn't used to war! At first, horror filled his imagination and temporarily numbed his responses. But not for long. The terror of the impending danger throbbed back like an anesthetic wearing off. He was king and every eye would look to him for leadership. How could he tell them that he had absolutely no idea what to do?

Anyone can walk with God in times of prosperity and peace. It's not hard to love when it's reciprocated. It's easy to be gracious with people who are loving and understanding. It's not difficult to believe when your faith isn't being sorely tested. However, what is our response when we go through the tough times? Will we trust God then? To show us His faithfulness and miracles of deliverance, we may have to confront some fierce challenges that literally bring us to our knees? We don't bow easily!

Jehoshaphat did on this occasion; he knew that prayer was his only option! He walked before the Living God, therefore he knew what to do in times of trouble: he *must* inquire of the Lord. He sent the word out to everyone to come and join him. Courageously, he stood before them and declared, "O Lord, God of our fathers, are You not the God who is in heaven? You rule over all the kingdoms of the nations. Power and might are in Your hand, and no one can withstand You." (A perfect start to any prayer!)

The moment we do this we access the grace of God. When we are threatened in any way; whether it's our lives, our marriages, our children, our health, our businesses, our church, or anything at all, it's imperative to make it our number one priority to seek the Lord. It changes everything. That's when the miracles happen!

As Jehoshaphat prayed, he recalled God's faithfulness to Israel and the past victories that were strewn throughout their history. He knew that God had given them the land where they lived. God had destroyed their enemies before and so he reasoned He would rescue them again. Infused with fresh confidence to rely once again upon God's goodness and mercy, he reaffirmed the prayer of previous generations when they'd said, "If calamity comes upon us, whether the sword of judgment, or plague or famine, we will stand in Your presence…and will cry out to You in our distress, and You will hear us and save us."

This is a great principle to remember when we are faced with a seemingly impossible situation. Think back over the many varied circumstances you've experienced that have been completely out of your control. Has God helped you in the past? Will He not help you again? Will His grace and power run out the more He uses them? Do the granaries of His mercy become depleted the more we draw upon them? It's impossible! God is never impoverished by giving! If we are smart, we will come to Him for help, again and again. Why ever not? The more we give Him opportunity to bless us, the more we will see of His love and faithfulness in our lives.

Jehoshaphat placed himself in a position for blessing. He had a living relationship with the covenant God of Israel. He hadn't any doubt that God would hear them when they called and would help them in their crisis. He had also worked out (without anyone telling him), that apart from divine intervention, they were all destined for a crushing defeat!

Aware of this, Jehoshaphat continued to pour out his heart to God. Not that prayer is telling God anything that He doesn't know already. He just loves it when we come to him and tell Him anyway! Jehoshaphat was totally honest about their predicament; "We don't have what it takes to defeat this army. We don't have the numbers; we don't have the power. In fact, we don't know what to do! But, our eyes are pinned on You." (We are safe when God fills our view!)

These words are music to God's ears. This is one prayer that attracts heaven's full attention. Divine help was ready, waiting in the wings. The Spirit of the Lord came upon a man called Jahaziel who prophesied and reassured them, "Do not be afraid or discouraged by this vast army. For the battle is not yours, but God's. Tomorrow, march down against them…You will not have to fight this battle. Take up your positions; stand firm and see the deliverance the Lord will give you…Do not be afraid; do not be discouraged. Go out and face them, and the Lord will be with you" (v15-17)).

Here was God's Word, right in their situation. He was going to take care of everything! They would not even have to fight; God was going into battle for them. It's amazing the strength that comes when we hear from God. It releases faith and annihilates fear, when naturally our hearts would faint.

The people gathered around Jehoshaphat. Some fell down, not because they were afraid. They worshiped! Others were so excited, they stood and praised the Lord with loud voices. God's Word had released faith and unclenched their fear. One minute they were so scared not knowing what to do – the next minute they were so full of joy, they couldn't contain themselves. No wonder! God was with them and He was going ahead of them. When they went to war the next day, they were shouting the victory before the battle had even begun! They had put away their swords and were warming up their vocal chords ready to sing. Each individual song merged together into one exhilarating chorus of victory. Gratitude began to gather momentum, culminating in a magnificent crescendo: "Give thanks to the Lord, for His love endures forever." Really? Whoever heard of such a strategy in warfare? It's certainly not common place, that's for sure!

However, something amazing happened in the heavenly realm, that caused a mighty commotion on the battlefield before they even arrived. God sent chaos and confusion into the enemy's ranks, so they began to slaughter each other. When Jehoshaphat and his army arrived, there were dead bodies everywhere. The battle was over; all they had to do was pick up the plunder. In fact, there was so much, it took them three days to carry it all away! The following day they all gathered together to thank God in the Valley of Beracah, which in Hebrew means "blessing." It certainly was!

Spiritual warfare with *singing*? Absolutely. It has been of great value for me personally. Week after week, month after month, and year after year, I have had the privilege of leading God's people in worship. It's been a wellspring of life and a fountain of joy. My little piece of earth has been totally transformed by touching heaven.

Yet, on other occasions, it has been a spiritual discipline to sing when I haven't always felt like it. But I'm so glad I did! In the healing atmosphere of God's presence, I have poured out my heart to Him. Tears have moistened my eyes as my emotions have emerged, and my fears have been washed away in the river of His grace. When you lift your gaze towards God and are engulfed in His love, you are fortified to face anything!

Jehoshaphat would never have experienced such an amazing miracle, if Israel's enemies had not come to fight against them. He would never have seen God's strength in contrast to his weakness. He would never have witnessed the extraordinary power of praise and worship! These were life-changing lessons money couldn't buy, as they are for us today!

God longs for us to know Him and trust Him; so He uses our individual circumstances to demonstrate His faithfulness. He shows His tenderness in comparison to our toughness. He manifests His mercy when we least expect it. He displays His kindness when we don't deserve it.

It's just called 'Grace' – God's undeserved kindness!

However, there may be certain times in our lives when we will be required to engage with our enemy. David's victory over Goliath is a classic illustration; a shepherd boy's fight against the notorious giant. David knew God: Many were the times the Lord had helped him rescue a little lamb from the jaws of a lion. He'd wrestled with bears to protect his father's sheep; even killed them when necessary. God had helped him in the past. He would help him now.

Deep-seated fury seethed inside him, and simmered over at the sight of this brutal enemy. How dare this towering bully intimidate God's people and traumatize them with such terror! He recognized the righteous indignation that rose within him. He had felt it when fighting for his flocks. Now a similar ferocity pulsated through his veins; God's people were under attack. All eyes were on him as he stepped out from the shadows of obscurity into the full light of day. No armor, no shield, no helmet or sword. Just a staff in his hand, a small pouch concealing five smooth stones from a nearby stream, and his sling was all he needed. God would do the rest!

Clothed with courage and filled with faith, David walked onto the battle field, and challenged his fierce and formidable opponent. "You come to me with sword, spear and javelin, but I come to you in the name of the Lord Almighty – the God of the armies of Israel, whom you have defied. Today the Lord will conquer you, and I will kill you and cut off your head…then I will give the dead bodies of your men to the birds and wild animals, and the whole world will know that there is a God in Israel. And everyone will know that the Lord does not need weapons to rescue His people. It is His battle, not ours. The Lord will give you to us!" (1 Samuel 17:45-47 NLT).

The rest is history. We know who won! Goliath's downfall was dramatic. Pride plummeted in spectacular fashion. David wasn't the least surprised even if everyone else was. One little well-aimed stone from a well-worn sling and God's enemy fell to the ground, fatally wounded. Fear was dealt a 'gigantic' death-blow on the battlefield that day. No one would have believed it unless they knew the God of Israel and His unusual ways of warfare! God doesn't look for might or strength. He doesn't require power or prestige. He just loves it when we trust Him!

David did, and the result was recorded forever!

There is one other option however. The Lord may deliver us by taking us out of this world to be with Him; 'The righteous pass away…And no one seems to care or wonder why. No one seems to understand that God is protecting them from the evil to come. For the godly who die will rest in peace' (Isaiah 57:1-2 NLT).

God knows our future; we don't, which is why we need to trust Him, especially when accidents happen suddenly, or loved ones die, seemingly prematurely. These are indeed profound mysteries, and really only find their answers in the all-wise and all-loving heart of God. We won't always understand, but we can rely on the One who knows exactly what He's doing, even if He doesn't explain to us the reasons why!

What is vitally important is that, in the light of any eventuality, we know where we are going to spend eternity! When we place our faith in God, we can confidently leave the outworking of our lives with Him.

In all these scenarios, one thing is sure: God is our deliverer. He either will deliver us *from* the battles that come against us, or He will deliver us *in the midst* of the battle, or He will take us *out* of the battle, when that time comes.

And our times are in His hands!

CHAPTER THIRTY-THREE

The Purpose of the Potter

There was a day when the Lord spoke to the prophet Jeremiah and instructed him to go down to the Potter's house. He was to watch closely. There was something God wanted him to see. The Potter was busy working. With firm hands, he cupped the formless clay and placed it on the wheel. What would he make out of such a hard lump of mud? Clearly, without his skillful touch, it would stay just as it was, cold and useless.

As Jeremiah watched the deft hands of the Potter, he noticed him abruptly hesitate. Stopping the wheel, he lifted the moistened clay and felt around it. He seemed to be searching for something. What could it be it? Maybe a gritty shard or a flaw in the material, which had marred the vessel he was making. Usually, rejects were tossed away and thrown into a bin with all the other rubbish. Not this time. The Potter patiently removed the blemish, splashed more water on the clay, squashed it back into a rough lump and started over again; pounding, pressing and gently prodding. Gradually the clay began to relax and soften, yielding to the perfect pressure of the Potter's creative genius. With increasing speed the wheel spun round, as the transformation began to take place

Jeremiah continued to watch, as the Potter's hands dug down deep into the center of the clay. With instinctive precision and equal passion, he purposefully remolded the vessel. Almost magically, it came to life. There before him was the most exquisitely shaped pot that he had ever seen.

For a moment, Jeremiah stood lost in the meanderings of his imagination. Ah! Now he could picture the final masterpiece; hand painted meticulously with striking strokes of color, finished off with touches of glistening gold, fit to adorn the Temple court or beautify the royal palace.

Jeremiah was jolted back to reality as the Lord's message came strongly to his heart; "Like clay in the hand of the Potter, so are you in my hand, O House of Israel" (Jeremiah 18:6). Now it made sense. What a perfect picture of hope! What a magnificent parable of the heavenly Potter remaking marred and broken lives. God was not going to reject His people because of their hardened hearts. He was going to remove the shards of disobedience and the grit of their rebellion, and reshape them according to His divine purpose.

This is what we are – God's clay pots! His workmanship. In 2 Corinthians 4:7 Paul writes, 'We have this treasure in jars of clay to show that this all-surpassing power is from God and not from us.' Each one of us is uniquely designed to display God's grace. As we yield our lives to His touch, He makes us into vessels of honor, that contain His glory, in the way that He knows is best! In *The Message* paraphrase of Romans 9:21 we read, 'Clay doesn't talk back to the fingers that mold it saying, "Why did you shape me like this?" Isn't it obvious that a potter has a perfect right to shape one lump of clay into a vase for holding flowers and another into a pot for cooking beans?' Good question!

God's designs and purposes are specific to each one of us. Will we trust Him, and stop comparing what He is doing in our lives to the work He's doing in others? The relevance of this could not have been more apparent and significant to me, than when I read about two amazing men from my own family history.

Two amazing men

A few years ago, Len and I returned to the UK for a holiday. In the course our travels, we visited the Arnos Vale Cemetery in the city of Bristol, England. My great-great-great-great grandfather, and great-great-great-great uncle are buried here. In the brochure, they are both mentioned as being 'noteworthy' but coach tours bring people to view one grave in particular – that of George Muller. (I'm honored to call him "Uncle George," because I am related to him by his marriage to my fourth great grandfather's sister.) Many have heard of him as being the man who cared for thousands of orphans in the same era as Charles Dickens. Nevertheless, the fact that God used him in such a public and powerful way, was no reflection of the young man he had been in his earlier years. The story of Muller's life is fascinating.

Apparently, he had no initial interest in Christianity. He was referred to as a 'Prussian playboy.' He enjoyed a luxurious lifestyle without having a penny to his name and consequently he was always dodging the debtors. Eventually though, his crimes caught up with him; at the age of sixteen he was locked up in a prison cell for three long weeks. His father made restitution for him by paying his debts and so he was released. But, on his return home, George was beaten severely in the hope that he would change his wicked ways. It didn't work! On his own admission, he remained as sinful in his heart as ever. (He was forever getting into trouble!)

Yet, the Lord had His hand upon this unique character. During his time studying at a German university, one of his friends invited him to a local Christian home fellowship. The meeting made a deep impression on Muller. In fact, it was the turning point in his life. He suddenly came to understand why Jesus died on the cross, bearing the punishment that should have been his. It was this revelation of Jesus love for him, that caused him to kneel by his bed and ask God to forgive his sins. This was the beginning of the rest of an amazing life. He decided to become a missionary.

About three years later, after he finished university, he traveled to England to join the London Missionary Society. It was while he was there that he heard of my great-great-great-great grandfather, Anthony Norris Groves, who was a wealthy dentist in Exeter. His story is also fascinating and brilliantly documented by Dr. Robert Dann in his book *Father of Faith Missions.*

In the early years of his life, Groves was deeply challenged to live by faith. He wrote a small tract called 'Christian Devotedness,' which encouraged the practice of giving away one's possessions to the poor instead of storing up treasures on earth. But, he didn't only write about it; he practiced what he preached. He and his wife began by giving away one tenth of his income, finding ways to help needy families in town. Eventually, they decided to reduce their expenses, and give away the rest of their money!

Later, at the age of 33, Groves sold their large house and gave a younger relative his £1,500 a-year dental practice. (A fortune in those days!) He then left England and set out with his wife and two little boys on a wildly dangerous journey to Baghdad, becoming the first missionaries in Iraq. They didn't have support from a church denomination (as they weren't ordained), neither did they have any personal financial security. They made the decision to depend upon the Lord alone for all their needs, which is exactly what they did.

George Muller was profoundly challenged by reading Grove's tract and hearing his story. Consequently, he rededicated his whole life to the Lord in complete surrender of heart. He said that the

271

change he experienced was 'like a second conversion.' Muller later acknowledged that this was a major pivotal turning point in his life.

However, his association with him would not stop there. It just so happened that during this time, Muller preached once a week at a small chapel in Exeter. On these occasions, he would lodge in a room of a local boarding school, that occupied a large house nearby. It also 'just so happened' that the young housekeeper who worked there was also the sister of the remarkable dentist, Anthony Norris Groves, who had been the previous owner!

Mary Groves shared her brother's devotion to Christ and his willingness to trust God in all things. It wasn't long before George and Mary fell in love and were married. From then on, the names of Groves and Muller were indelibly united, both by marriage and the call to missions. This is the connection I have with both these amazing men of God. However, their lives turned out so differently. Visiting their grave sites made this even more glaringly apparent.

George Muller's final resting place was placed in a prominent position next to a well-trodden footpath, where people could linger and read the epitaph on the impressive gravestone. Now, here were Len and I, standing right beside his memorial headstone. Silently and somberly, I slowly read the inscription on the massive marble monument. I will never forget the emotion of that moment. The impact carved its imprint deeply upon my heart, as I took in the following words:

In loving memory of George Muller

Founder of the Ashley Down Orphanage

Born September 27, 1805

Fell asleep March 10, 1898

He trusted in God with whom nothing shall be impossible

And in His Beloved Son Jesus Christ our Lord who said,

'I go unto my Father, and whatsoever you shall ask in my name

That will I do, that the Father may be glorified in the Son.'

And in His inspired word which declares that

'All things are possible to him that believeth.'

And God fulfilled these declarations in the experience

Of his servant by enabling him to provide and care

For about 10,000 orphans.

~~

This memorial was erected by the spontaneous and

Loving gifts of many of these orphans.

~~

During Muller's life, ten thousand orphans were taken into his care! In the 1800's, such children who had lost their parents had to beg, borrow or steal, just to survive. They were left to scavenge the streets like vermin, so the government placed them in 'poorhouses' where they worked long and arduously in the cruelest of conditions. Muller began to pray about starting an orphan house himself, where no child would be turned away due to poverty or race. They would all be educated and trained for a trade. He trusted that God would supply all their needs, which He did! Part of his incredible testimony was how the Lord provided the equivalent of $129,000,000 during his life to accommodate and care for these impoverished children, when he only had two shillings (50cents) in his pocket to start with! For sixty years, the orphans had homes and shelter, were clothed and fed, and never went without one meal!

Len and I only had time to see one of these massive homes he had built, and there were four others! Our jaws almost scraped the ground as we stood there incredulous at its size alone. The blocks of granite stone towered imposingly above us. The extensive walls stretched out like welcoming arms that had protected thousands of vulnerable waifs and strays in their embrace. It was breathtaking.

There was another reason why founding the orphanages was so important to Muller. He wanted to demonstrate that God is real. This was to be his enduring legacy. He had proved God in his own life and wanted others to share the same experience.

In 1835, he felt impressed to embark on the adventure of his life! He wrote in his journal "Now, if I, a poor man, simply by prayer and faith, obtained ***without asking any individual*** the means for establishing and carrying on an Orphan-House: there would be something which, with the Lord's blessing, might be instrumental in strengthening the faith of the children of God, …whereby it may be seen that God is ***faithful still and hears prayers still.***"

The five impressive structures he built (covering 13 acres over Ashley Downs), still stand today as evidence of the faithfulness of Muller's God. Since then, houses 1 and 3 have been converted into many individual units, but a plaque on the wall still gives credit to 'George Muller of Bristol.' Houses 2, 4 and 5 are now occupied by the City of Bristol College. Even so, the legacy of Muller's faith still shines as a beacon today inspiring Christians to believe in the power of prayer and God's Word. What lessons of sacrifice and surrender! What an incredible testimony of a man so greatly influenced by my ancestral grandfather, Anthony Norris Groves.

Later, Len and I looked around for his gravesite, assuming it would be similar to that of George Muller's. After all, they are both listed as 'notable' people buried in the Arnos Vale Cemetery. In vain we searched up and down the narrow paths. Why couldn't we find it? According to the brochure, we knew it was here somewhere.

Quite disheartened, we very nearly gave up, but before leaving, we thought of one last possibility. I went to the office staff to ask for their help. It would cost £30 for a search map to find the exact spot. Nevertheless, they warned us it wouldn't be easy to find. The foliage in that area was heavily overgrown and almost impossible to penetrate.

But we were not going to be deterred! I had come all the way from Australia to stand by his grave. I had only just finished reading the amazing story of Grove's venerable life of faith on the mission fields. It was legendary! So why was his grave buried under so many

275

weeds and not on display for everyone to see? Didn't he also have an impressive marble headstone? We were totally perplexed!

We handed over another £20 to hire one of the gravediggers to tear away the thick undergrowth and find the location. Forty-five minutes later, there it was, hidden many meters from the footpath, mantled with a cloak of moss and wet debris. What a vivid contrast between the two graves! Both were the earthly resting places of two wonderful men of God. One remembered and honored. The other, seemingly forgotten.

I reached for my little penknife attached to my key ring, knelt down by the freshly uncovered plot and scraped away the mud that concealed the markings. I was so thrilled to discover the engravings that had been obscured for so long. Some had worn away over the years, but as each letter became visible the words became clearer:

"Thy words were found and I ate them, and
Your word was unto me the joy and rejoicing
of my heart, for I am called by thy name,
O Lord of Hosts."
(Jeremiah 15:16 KJV)

Here it was! Oh, the wonder of that moment as I imbibed the wonder of my new discovery. I had been deeply moved by reading his biography before we came, so I felt as if I had journeyed with him through his many struggles and heartaches. It was *his* writings that had inspired the great George Muller, and yet *his* life turned out so differently. He and his wife had given away all their possessions, and struggled financially for the rest of their lives. They worshiped the same God as Muller, but He was to take them on completely different paths.

Tragedy became a close traveling companion to Groves. Even before he and his wife had left England to go overseas, their little five-year-old daughter became very ill and died soon after. One of their friends remarked, "The loss of their only daughter was used as a means by which they became yet more separate from the earth, and while it made their path clear (to follow their missionary call), it strengthened them to devote themselves to God." What amazing commitment they showed at that time, when many others may have crumbled!

When they did eventually set sail for Persia, they had to brave a massive storm. Then after disembarking, they rode over land in two large horse-drawn carriages. The wheels broke a few times and once the axle caught fire. The further east they journeyed, the roads became rougher and the inns where they stayed became dirtier. Two of their horses were stolen and two of them died. Sometimes, their carriages became stuck in mud for hours; other times they traveled in crude wagons with no springs. They endured nightmare periods of torrential rains, dangerous thieves and savage dogs. Bandits drew daggers at them without any provocation. Their journey lasted six months, over 5,000 miles, most of which was through mountainous

277

terrain, across sandy deserts, over impassable roads and on unmade tracks of rocks and soggy soil. But the Lord protected them all.

When they arrived in Baghdad, Groves saw an opportunity to set up a mission school in the lower basement of their house. They started by teaching colloquial Arabic to the local children and then a few families asked for English lessons, seeing this as an entrance into the sphere of British influence in the East. Initially, forty-three boys and two girls attended. The school grew, giving them many opportunities to share the gospel, but times were uncertain for this brave little band of missionaries. Unfortunately, war threatened. So did cholera and the plague.

On March 28th, 1831, Groves wrote in his journal "The plague has entered this unhappy city." Sadly, they had to make the painful decision to close their fledgling school. No longer was it feasible to gather eighty children from the different parts of the city, without exposing them all to danger.

During the first turbulent two weeks, 7,000 people died out of a population of 75,000. Eventually, between 1,500 and 2,000 were dying each day in the city of Baghdad alone. In just one month, the death toll was 30,000 with no apparent end in sight. The horrors and dangers of that time defy description. The basics of water and provisions became scarce, almost to the point of semi-starvation. However, Groves and his wife continued to place their trust solely in the Lord. Mary often spoke about the peace she had experienced since being in Baghdad, and the evidence of God's loving care. "We came out trusting only under His wing, and He will never forsake us." God never left them for one minute. Neither did their trials.

Each day they watched, as plague-ravaged bodies were carried out from the houses along the alleyway, on the opposite side of the street. From one end of the city to the other, the dead were brought to be buried in one mass common grave. If that wasn't enough, the Tigris river burst its banks and rose to a higher level than anyone could remember. More than half of the poorly constructed houses collapsed into the floodwaters. Floating debris and decaying flesh swept along the drains, submerging the graves and rubbish dumps.

The plague continued to wrap its cruel tentacles around the city. Many entire families were destroyed. In some homes, only one or two remained. Groves wrote in his journal, "But I hear of none save our own where death has not entered." So, it was devastating when only one week later, his wife became dangerously ill. He had felt sure the Lord would spare their family. He was left to conclude that "...His ways are not our ways, nor His thoughts our thoughts." (So true!)

Cholera was a fearsome diagnosis indeed, but the plague was a word that struck terror into all that heard it. The intense pain of the red oval swellings in the groin, armpits and neck was followed by delirium and death. With a severe headache and great difficulty in opening her eyes, Mary did her best to comfort her discouraged husband. (Aren't women great!) "I marvel at the Lord's dealing, but not more than at my own peace in such circumstances."

It was so hard for Groves to watch his wife suffer without being able to do anything to help her. Even God did not appear to be responding to their desperate cries. Seven days after Mary's first symptoms of the plague appeared, she quietly passed away. What made the sting even worse was the fact she died on the very day the shops reopened and the locals returned to work. Vegetables were seen on the streets again and drinking water came back down again to its normal price. The plague had passed. They had come so close to escaping it!

What a shock for those left behind to bear this loss. Mary had been such an incredible strength to all who knew her. Now she too had gone. Her body was wrapped in a sheet, laid on a flimsy frame of palm branches tied with cords on the back of a horse, and taken away for burial by two strangers. No one followed her remains to the grave, and no funeral rites were performed there. It would only have exposed the rest of her family to greater risk of infection. To this day, no one knows where she is buried.

Groves understandably struggled with loneliness and despair during this time. He thought how easy it had been to appear as an outstanding Christian with such a loving wife, a comfortable home, a rewarding profession and a stimulating circle of godly friends; and how hard it had been to maintain any Christian spirit at all when stripped bare and exposed to a thousand weaknesses. He regretted that at times he had been painfully slow to kiss the hand that had wounded him, and bless the hand that had poured out such sorrow.

Mercifully, he didn't wallow for long in the 'pit of despair' before grasping the lifeline of hope again. He marveled, "The sense of my Father's love and Savior's sympathy has never been taken from me amidst all my trials."

Three months after his wife passed away, their little baby also died. This was a double-barreled blow, beyond words. Groves was so grateful Mary didn't live to experience the final grief and loss that only parents who have lost a child would understand. A poignant entry in his journal reads, "The Lord took her (Mary) from the evil to come, and now has taken the dear little object of her love to her. Four of us are gone, and three are left." (This could almost have been a nineteenth century Job scenario!) Groves had greatly desired to blaze a burning trail on the mission field, as a testimony to the faithfulness of God. Surely now, he must have felt that the fire had fizzled into the tiniest flicker.

Both George Muller and Anthony Norris Groves were saved by the Lord and called into full-time service. Both placed the same trust in God's faithfulness. Both prayed fervently. One built notable buildings where thousands of orphans found refuge, and recorded miracle after miracle of God's loving care. The other wasn't able to leave such grandiose monuments and document such awe-inspiring stories. Even Grove's own house collapsed, as local floods seeped into the foundations of the basement floor. He suffered loss after tragic loss and felt himself to be a complete failure at the end of his life! He was even unable to pay for his own humble grave. George Muller bought his gravesite for him – the one we stood beside! How sad that he never knew the incredible impact his life and faith would have on so many, throughout the years. He will one day!

I have used these two illustrations from my own family line as examples of the different ways God shapes our lives to fulfill His purposes. We all have our own stories to tell. I have shared part of mine. But then, you have yours.

May I lovingly encourage you to trust that everything you are going through will be well worth it. More than you know! You have been saved for the praise of God's glorious grace. There will never be a greater honor or privilege.

Right now though, you may feel as if you are buried under a hundred tons of rock and the weight of the world is crushing down on you. But remember, it is the immense, unrelenting pressure of the earth upon the carbon crystal that finally forms the diamond. One day, we will thank God for the seasons of suffering that have pressed, buffed, cut and polished us. He is shaping us perfectly and fashioning us purposefully, because we are His…

… 'Diamonds in the Dark.'

~~

Len's Perspective

I loved Heather before I knew her! She existed as a dream in my heart, even when I was young. So, when we met, I felt I already knew her. I wrote this poem during the infancy of our relationship, as our love began to blossom and flourish throughout our forty years of marriage, my feelings haven't changed. In fact, my dream has become the most wonderful reality, and our love continues to grow.

"I have always known you."   Len Magee 1976

I knew you once when you were only a dream.

An idea that flit through my mind as winged lightning;

A warm thought that spiraled away

Into endless, empty blackness.

I clutched at you, though you were never far away.

And I despaired.

Would your reality ever emerge to conquer me?

Some said you didn't

Or couldn't,

Or wouldn't exist.

The ideal, I confess, more than once faded,

Grew sick and pale,

Just a long, lost moment of childish joy.

Gone forever?

All the time you were hidden in God's garden

Among the spices and growing with the leaves of laughter,

Planted in the warm fertile soil of surprises

Until, sent forth by the Dove of Joy,

You timidly, tenderly blushed my way,

And like the jeweled dawning of a new day

You arrived, sun crusted in dazzling dew.

When I saw you,

You hesitated, stopped and smiled, half shy.

With an impish wink, you tossed your head,

Turned your back and walked on

And your mind ran away,

And for the first time – you let it go.

Your girlish weakness

Was the strength that hooked my soul.

You stood as the Bethlehem Star,

Moved and drew me

As a fascinated, stumbling child.

Drunk with the power of your confidence – I followed.

We bathed in our love-song

And skipped as spring lambs in our excitement.

Your voice alone put its feet up and basked

In the burning fireplace of my soul.

Precious was its gentle whisper in my ears.

Precious were the honeyed thoughts I saw within your tears.

And our spirits ran together as a flood of silver light,

Snapped shut, and interlocked in a band of steel.

All the worlds fiction

Would never fill one sentence of your reality,

For though I knew you once when you were but a dream,

Now I know

I have always known you.

~~

There was something else I knew beyond a shadow of a doubt; it was God that sovereignly drew us together. There's an incredible strength that accompanies that knowing. It has fortified us in the toughest of storms. It has reassured us in the most cyclonic winds that have come against us. Marriage doesn't guarantee that life will be perfect. It won't be. Love can hurt! Especially when the one you love is suffering. But it does means you can pray and encourage one another in the experiences of life. We've laughed until we've cried, and cried until we've laughed.

When I learned that Heather had been diagnosed with Type 1 diabetes, I remember parking my car on the side of the road and crying like a baby. (I could because I was traveling by myself on that occasion.) It broke my heart! However, I was with Heather when they confirmed her diagnosis of breast cancer. I didn't cry then. How could I? She needed me to be strong and supportive, not

285

drown in a pool of tears in front of her. To be honest, I really didn't comprehend what was happening. It was all so foggy. Our world was suddenly unraveling before our eyes. What could I do? Flitting through my mind were a million thoughts. Every now and then, I felt as if I was all out at sea and there were dangerous rocks ahead. At times, I felt spiritually seasick.

I knew it wasn't all about me. In a sense, what enabled us to get through this was although it was about Heather, it was primarily about God. His will, His ways and above all, His glory. However, Heather has asked me briefly to explain how I felt then, and how I feel now.

I have seen firsthand just how devastating it has been for her to have such a confronting diagnosis and how difficult it was for her to face the operation that would seek to rob her, not only of her womanhood and femininity, but rip into her soul in a very profound and mystical way.

Most men, if they are honest, have experienced overwhelming love and joy in this particular aspect of their marriage. The Lord tells us through the writings of King Solomon in Proverbs 5:19 (*The Message*), 'Enjoy the wife you married as a young man! Lovely as an angel, beautiful as a rose – don't ever quit taking delight in her body. Never take her love for granted!' The NIV says; 'May you always be satisfied and ravished by her love.'

Sure I hurt, but she hurt more. But, God has given us both His grace as we have gone through this devastating experience together.

He has enabled us to come to terms with the situation. Life is what it is! Thankfully though, there are many more important issues in our lives, and these are what we have chosen to focus on.

Finally, I am strengthened and energized by my beliefs. A. W. Tozer once said 'all of life is theological.' Theology simply means 'knowledge of God.' The Bible and God's promises are real to me. They are rock solid and they work! They make a difference in my life and marriage. Without the Lord, I would not have known His loving grace and strength which has enabled me to support Heather through her cancer and recovery.

Ah, but then I would never have had the privilege to meet and marry her in the first place. When we married, our commitment to each other was "for better or for worse." Sometimes life is better. Sometimes it's amazing! Sometimes it's worse. Then sometimes, all of a sudden, it seems to get a lot worse! But, there aren't only two of us in our marriage! There are three! The Bible tells us that a 'triple braided cord is not easily broken' (Ecclesiastes 3:12 NLT), and that third strand is the strongest–God! He has not only held us together, but strengthened our love. His love never fails!

I pray we will always trust Him in everything we go through, and never doubt His love!

Author's Update

Last year, I had my latest reconstruction surgery. Since then there have developed further complications. I had been told I no longer needed to attend the oncology clinic. However, it looks like I must return once more! I have just been diagnosed with multiple squamous cell skin cancers! Round 3 coming up! Another shock, yet another opportunity to draw strength from the reservoirs of God's fathomless love and faithfulness.

If we ever meet, you may notice my latest battle scars. Some battles we will fight…and win. Others we may not. (We'll ultimately win either way!) Let's keep fighting the real fight…the fight of faith!

Meanwhile, Matts recovery is still a work in progress. During the last few years, we have seen some amazing breakthroughs, but we have still to find the last few elusive pieces of this intricate puzzle before the picture is complete. He is still in the process of 'enduring' through the complexities of his challenging illness. However, that's another story for another book maybe. But that is for him to write!

Life is what it is and as a family, we are learning to embrace it, whether we like it or not! Notice, I did say 'learning! However, the question the Lord asked Matt is indelibly imprinted on my heart, and is pertinent to us all; "Will you trust Me, no matter what?"

By God's grace, we will!

APPENDIX

Can Christians be Under a Curse?

This is an interesting question. (I'm so glad you asked!) The Bible makes it quite clear that when sin entered the world, so did the curse. That's where sickness comes from. That's why we die. We have all been infected by the sin virus. Suffering and death are temporary intruders into a once perfect creation. They will be done away with eventually. At this moment though, we are still left with their devastating effects. The whole creation is 'groaning as in the pain of childbirth right up to this present time' (Romans 8:22).

Although we all live and breathe in a cursed world, it's great to know that Christ will one day restore our bodies and the whole of creation to perfection! This is the glorious hope of all who have been born again by the Holy Spirit. We have been saved through believing that Jesus died for us. He took our place, our punishment and our death so that we would never again have to experience the effects of the curse!

That being understood, let's now consider the suggestion that a child of the living God can be under a personal curse (as opposed to the general curse).

In the Old Testament, the Hebrew words for curse (according to Lawrence Richards Expository Dictionary of Bible Words) are 'arar' (meaning to bind or render powerless) and 'qalal' (meaning the loss or withdrawal of a blessing, which God longed for His people to enjoy). Curses were the result of God's judgment on His people if they didn't obey His commands (Deuteronomy 28:20-45). Blessings and curses were intrinsic to the Law of Moses. However, we are not subject to that 'Law' anymore. Jesus paid the penalty for all our sin and law-breaking, once and for all when He died on the cross, and has blessed us more than we ever deserved.

The definition of a curse (from the Oxford Dictionary) is: 'A solemn utterance intended to invoke a supernatural power to inflict harm or punishment on someone or something.' In the light of this, the idea of a Christian living under a personal curse poses a serious problem for me. In the same way that God cannot justify me and condemn me at the same time, neither can He bless me and curse me simultaneously. I have been set free! What from? God has saved me from Satan's tyranny, which he had a legal right to exercise over me before Jesus rescued me from his grasp. I am eternally loved by God. Therefore, if a curse is an appeal to a supernatural power to inflict evil destruction or punishment on me, that request must first receive God's authorization. Because Jesus is Lord, He has the final word. Thankfully!

Remember Job

In the account of Job we read that Satan was not allowed to do anything to him without God's express permission. In fact, it was God who drew Satan's attention to the amazing man Job was. Satan sneered in disbelief, insinuating that God's friend only loved Him because he'd been so blessed. To prove this was not the case, it was God Himself who gave consent for Job to be tested (not cursed) by the enemy.

If Job went to some churches today, he might possibly be told he was under a curse of the devil and needed prayer for deliverance from demonic powers! Nevertheless, all the prayers of God's people would not have made the slightest difference in Job's dire situation. Neither did the condemning counsel from his friends; "You must have sinned…your children must have sinned…God is punishing you…you are a hypocrite. . .you need to repent for you are a wicked man!" Oh, isn't that just what a suffering person needs to hear! Job was struggling enough in coming to terms with the combined losses of his children, his wealth, his servants, his cattle, his possessions and health. Then his friends hammer him spiritually to cap off his problems nicely. Thank you so much! They assumed suffering was the direct consequence of sin, and that divine favor was evidenced by a man's good health and material prosperity. They were so full of their own views and opinions, that they thought any disagreement to their judgements was like resisting God Himself! So, in their tiresome tirades and long-drawn-out speeches, they set out to prove that God always rewarded good and punished evil in this present life.

Job's friends gave him no helpful answer at all. Not one! They just made him feel a whole lot worse. No wonder God was so angry with them. They had misrepresented Him in such a damaging way, and misunderstood the real reason why Job was going through such trials. In fact, his so-called friends almost did more harm to Job's soul than the devil himself!

Unfortunately, Job's comforters can still be found today. They use the same arguments to justify people's pain, not understanding how these views totally undermine what Jesus accomplished for us on the cross, devalue the cost of our salvation, and detract from the reality that we have been saved and set free!

When people don't have a functional and practical theology of suffering, weakness or failure, they are unable to see that God is actually working in their lives through their trials. Consequently, they have to blame something or someone. Generational curses are one explanation some people use to explain sickness and suffering. Surely, God wants the best for us, therefore how could affliction be a blessing to anyone? Quickly they conclude that the child of God who is experiencing distress, must evidently have very little faith or it must be God's judgment upon them in some way.

How is this remotely feasible? Being a Christian means that we have been born into God's family. He is now our Heavenly Father and we are His children. We have been purchased by Jesus death on the cross. He became a curse *for* us. Galatians 3:13 says, 'Christ redeemed us from the curse of the law by becoming a curse for us.' He redeemed us to bless us! God will never be angry with us again. He cannot love us any more than He does already. Jesus said, "As the Father has loved me, so have I loved you" (John 15:9). Neither can He love us any less. God loves us in the same way He loves and delights in His Son. How amazing is this!

So, if a curse is as an appeal to a supernatural power to inflict harm or punishment upon someone, why would we think that God would allow us to be cursed, when we are the focus of His eternal and everlasting love?

If anyone should have been cursed, it would have been Peter. He called down curses on himself repeatedly when he denied even knowing Jesus (Mark 14:71). Yet we are never told that a curse came on him. In fact, it was Peter who Jesus singled out to care for His sheep. He was the disciple who preached on the Day of Pentecost, when about 3,000 people believed his message and were baptized. Acts 2:43 says, 'Everyone was filled with awe, and many wonders and miraculous signs were done by the apostles.' Peter was one of those apostles. Was this evidence of someone who was under a curse? On the contrary!

As Christians, we are beneficiaries of God's blessings – not God's curses! This is what God's Word says about us:

1)   2 Corinthians 5:17. 'Therefore, if anyone is in Christ, he is a new creation; the old has gone, the new has come!' What a wonderful reality. When we became part of God's family, the umbilical cord that tied us to our past was severed. We haven't just been reassembled; we've been re-created! We have been given an entirely new nature. Do we carry over curses into our brand-new life?

2)   1 Corinthians 3:16. 'Don't you know that you yourselves are God's temple and God's Spirit lives in you?' Mark 3:25 says; 'If a house is divided against itself, that house cannot stand.' Can curses cohabit with blessings in the temple of the Living God?

3)   Ephesians 2:6. 'And God has raised us up with Christ and seated us with Him in the heavenly realms.' This is the best place to see life from God's perspective! Can we be cursed at the same time as being exalted with Christ, in such an elevated, out-of-reach position?

4)   Colossians 2:10. We are complete in Him (NKJV). I love this word 'complete.' The dictionary defines it as 'finished, ended, concluded, done, accomplished, settled, absolute, perfect!' God has cancelled the debt we owed and paid the price for our sin. In 2 Corinthians 5:21(NLT) we read, 'For God made Christ, who never sinned, to be the offering for our sin, so that we could be made right with God, through Christ.' How amazing! Could a curse even get oxygen in the atmosphere of 'complete'?

5)   1 John 3:1. We are children of God and He is our Heavenly Father. Are we better parents than He is? Would we put a curse on our children if they did something wrong? I hope not! Then, if it was in our power, would we not stop others from cursing them also! So why would we expect any less from God?

6)   Ephesians 1:3 (NLT). We have been 'blessed with every spiritual blessing in the heavenly realms because we belong to Christ.' No mention of curses! Even when Balaam was asked to curse Israel by their enemies (Numbers 22-24), he was clearly told by God not even to think about it! What? Curse the people He loved? No way! "You must not put a curse on those people because they are blessed!" But the temptation was huge. Balaam just had to name his price! Gold, silver,

fame and fortune. All for just for one curse. However, God did not allow him! In fact, an angel with a drawn sword stood right in his way! He got the message. "How can I curse those whom God has not cursed? I have received a command to bless: He has blessed and I cannot change it." Here it is in black and white! In Romans 8:31 and 33, Paul asks, 'If God is for us, who can be against us?' 'Who will bring any charge against those whom God has chosen?' Great question!

7) Galatians 3:13. 'Christ redeemed us from the curse of the law by becoming a curse for us.' In Galatians 3:3, Paul describes observing the law as 'human effort.' Under the old covenant, the children of Israel came under judgments and curses if they were disobedient. So why did God give the law when He knew they couldn't possibly keep His commandments? It was to reveal their sinfulness and show how much they needed a Savior to deliver them. Breaking the law brought curses. But we are not under the law. We are now under grace!

8) Ephesians 1:6. God has made us 'accepted in the beloved' (KJV). In the New Testament, Christians are often described as 'Beloved.' This word highlights the amazing love God has for us. Ephesians 1:7-8 amplifies this by saying, 'In Him we have redemption through His blood, the forgiveness of sins, in accordance with the riches of God's grace that He lavished

upon us with all wisdom and understanding.' Could curses be conceived in the womb of such extravagant love?

9)   Hebrews 10:14. We have been 'made perfect forever,' and now 'glorified' (Romans 8:30). What is it about 'perfected' we don't understand? When Jesus shared the Last Supper with His disciples before He died, He told them He was making a new covenant with them and it would be sealed by His blood, which meant that the old covenant was about to be made redundant. Finished. Passed it's 'used-by date!' Gone forever. It was going to be replaced by a brand new one. Curses were never included in God's new covenant with us.

10)   Matthew 28:18. Before Jesus returned to heaven, He made an incredible statement; He told His disciples, "All authority in heaven and earth has been given unto Me." This universal dominion has been conferred upon Him by God. He has all power. He holds 'the keys of hell and death' (Revelation 1:18 KJV), which means that Satan doesn't! God has enthroned Him as the 'King of kings and the Lord of lords' (1 Timothy 6:15). He has been given 'the name that is above every name' (Philippians 2:9). There will never be a greater authority. So, if an appeal made to the highest supernatural power for us to be cursed, do you think that God, who loves us so much, would grant that request for one moment? I think not!

11) Ephesians 1:13-14. When we believed in Christ, God marked us 'with a seal, the promised Holy Spirit, who is a deposit guaranteeing our inheritance…' A deposit is given in advance as a secure down payment. We have been sealed by the Holy Spirit. We have been set apart unto God Himself. This has incredible implications for us now. We are perfectly safe and secure. Can a curse possibly pass through God's impenetrable seal?

12) Romans 4:7 'Blessed *and* happy *and* to be envied are those whose iniquities are forgiven and whose sins are covered up *and* completely buried' (AMP). Would you envy anyone who was cursed? We have been given the greatest gift ever! The fact we've been forgiven means that curses suffocate in the grave where our sins are buried!

So, in the penetrating light of these verses alone, is our son Matt under a curse because he's been ill for so long? Am I under a curse because I've had cancer? Was my husband under a curse because he suffered a stroke some years ago? Is our family under a curse because we have gone through so many trials during the last few years? Absolutely not! The cross says it all! The extent to which Jesus demonstrated His love for us, removes any questions about us being under a personal curse.

Perfect love casts out all fear!

Perhaps, to complete this section, we should consider who Jesus is to those who belong to Him. He has been given the name above all names. There are several of His names that show how safe we are.

1) Jesus is called our 'Shield' (2 Samuel 22:31).

William Gurnall in his book *The Christian in Complete Armour* reminds us that the shield is not for the defense of any specific part of the body like the other pieces are; the helmet for the head; the plate for the breast. The shield is intended for the protection of the whole body, so it is vast and long. It was made to defend the soldier in the fierce combat of battle, diverting poisoned arrows and cushioning heavy blows from the enemy. The Lord acts as our shield from the lies and accusations of our adversary. He stands between us and the onslaught from our avid accuser. We hide behind His protective cover.

2) Jesus is called our 'Savior' (Luke 1:47).

We have been 'saved!' The Greek word is 'sozo' and is used in relation to our past, present and future! The definition in Strong's Concordance of the Bible is, 'delivered, protected, healed and made whole.' It doesn't get more watertight than that. Proverbs 26:2 makes it clear that 'an undeserved curse does not come to rest.' The cross deletes the curse once we are in Christ! Jesus is our Deliverer. It is interesting that one meaning of the word 'deliver' means 'to

APPENDIX

strike a blow as in delivering a punch.' Jesus death on the cross was the greatest power-punch ever delivered to Satan, in order to deliver us from his malevolent grip. God has 'delivered and drawn us to Himself out of the control and the dominion of darkness and has transferred us into the kingdom of the Son of His love, in Whom we have our redemption…(which means) the forgiveness of our sins' (Colossians 1:13, 14 AMP).

3) Jesus is called our 'Fortress' (Psalm 18:2).

The Psalmist often had to escape from his enemies, hiding in caves amongst the craggy rocks and fleeing to the mountains. He likens God to such places of concealment and security. When we are overwhelmed, Jesus is our refuge and strong tower (Psalm 61:3), the place where we can run to and find protection.

Fort Knox is known to be the most secure fortresses in the world. Built on multiple layers of cement and capped by 10 feet of solid graphite, it is impenetrable from below ground. The site was purposely located many miles inland, 430 feet above sea level (no danger of flooding), protected by mountains and surrounded by armed sentinels. Constant surveillance cameras cover every square inch. Tinted bullet-proof windows protect the well-kept secret of where the gold is secured. Behind the thick granite walls (reinforced by 750 tons of steel), are armed guards and a maze of locked doors. A 22-ton door firmly fastens the ultimate safe, with a combination number known only to ten members of staff. But each of them are

302

privy to just a small section of the complete sequence of numbers so they all must be present at any one time to open the vault. Inside, smaller chambers still have to be unlocked before the 4.582 metric tons (147.3 million ounces) of gold bullion can finally be accessed! This is one secure garrison!

What an illustration of Jesus our fortress. Hidden in Him we are completely safe!

More than Fort Knox safe!

4) Jesus is called 'The Lord, strong and mighty' (Psalm 24:8).

He is the Lord God Almighty (Revelation 4:8), the Lord of Hosts; the Commander of the armies of heaven! The angels bow before Him and obey His every word. 'Who is the King of glory?' the Psalmist asks and then answers his own rhetorical question, 'The Lord strong and mighty, the Lord invincible in battle…He is the King of glory' (Psalm 24:8,10 NLT). 'The Lord has made the heavens His throne; from there He rules over everything. (Psalm 103;19 NLT). God holds the scepter of His sovereignty and the orb of His authority over the whole world. Spurgeon says that God's 'matchless sovereignty is the pledge of our security and the pillar upon which our confidence may safely lean.' I love that! In every battle or conflict we are in, the Lord is with us. No one has ever pitted themselves against God and won! He is mighty. He is strong. He rules! His throne is established firmly in heaven, and from there

He decrees His plan and purposes for our lives. He has the last word, not our enemy!

This is not a comprehensive list by any means. I have just included a few of the names of Jesus that can help fortify us in our struggles. Understanding these truths has been so liberating for me. I trust they are for you too.

Let's live in the freedom for which Christ has set us free. Let's stand fast in that freedom, knowing who we are in Christ and who He is in us. Let's delight in His love for us and live to love Him in return.

Credits

My love and thanks to my husband Len and our children, Matt and Hannah, who have endured both the events in this story and the writing of the book! Legends!

Thanks also to Pastor Ken Legg and Len, for helping to edit and carefully review the theological aspects expressed in this book, and Lesley Wells (my sister-in-law) for editing and proofreading.

Thanks to my friend Steve Nugent, who has graciously helped me through the technical maze in producing these pages.

Thanks to my friend Paul Metcalfe for the photograph of the diamonds on the back cover.

Thank you also to my friend Kimbra Ochsner for sharing her typing skills in helping edit and prepare this book for print.

Thanks to my family and friends who have shown their love in a million and one different ways. Each one of you are incredibly special to me.

Thank you to our church for loving and supporting us through all our trials. Thank you to every one of you who have walked along side us, even when it looked like we might not survive. We have! It is all glory to our wonderful God who we serve together.

Thank you to Shanene Higgins, who has published this book. Working with her has been an honor and privilege.

To each and every one of you…thank you so much. I am and will remain eternally grateful.

Resources for further reading:

1) Explore the Book. Sidlow Baxter.

   Marshal Morgan and Scott. ©1951

2) There's no place Like Hope. Vickie Gerrard ©2004

3) The Christian in Complete Armour. William Gurnell.

   © 1864 Banner of Truth Trust.

4) The Five Silent Years of Corrie ten Boom.

   Pamela Rosewell Moore.

   © 1986 Zondervan.

5) Suffering and the Sovereignty of God. John Piper.

   ©2006 Crossways Books

6) Future Grace. John Piper.

   ©1995 Multnomah.

7) Buried Treasure. Victoria Finlay.

   ©2006 Sceptre (Hodd)

8) When God Weeps. Joni Eareckson Tada and Steven Estes.

   Copyright ©1997 Use by permission of Zondervan.

   www.zondervan.com

9) Streams in the Desert. Mrs. Charles Cowman.

   ©1944 Marshall Pickering.

10) Father of Faith Missions:

    The Life and Times of Anthony Norris Groves.

    Robert Dann ©2004 Authentic Media.

11) Pilgrim's Progress. John Bunyan. (1678) Public domain.

12) Through Gates of Splendor. Elizabeth Elliot.

©1956 Tindale House Publishers Inc. Wheaton, Illinois.

13) Singing in the Fire. Faith Cook.

©1995 The Banner of Truth Trust.

14) George Muller Delighted in God! Roger Steer.

©1981 Harold Shaw Publishers.

15) Praying Through Cancer. Susan Sorensen & Laura Geist.

©2006 W Publishing Group.

16) Mrs. C.H. Spurgeon. Charles Ray (Essex: Passmore & Alabaster, 1903) 81-82. (Public Domain.)

17) Faith's Checkbook. A Treasury of Daily Devotionals by C.H. Spurgeon. (Public Domain).

18) Expository Dictionary of Bible Words.

Lawrence O. Richards.

©1985 by the Zondervan Corporation. Grand Rapids, Michigan.

Biblical quotations

All scripture quotations, unless otherwise indicated, are taken from The HOLY BIBLE, New International Version®. NIV ® Copyright © 2011, by Biblica, Inc.™ Used by permission of Zondervan. All rights reserved worldwide. www.zondervan.com The "NIV" and "New International Version" are trademarks registered in the United States Patent and Trademark Office by Biblica, Inc.

Index

313

X

About the Author

Heather was born on September 14, 1956. She was the eldest of three sisters and grew up in a loving Christian family in England. She trained to be a teacher at Gypsy Hill College in Kingston, Surrey (not far from Wimbledon, where the English tennis finals are held each year).

It was during her final year at college that she met Len Magee, who was one of Britain's most loved gospel singers at that time. As the prayer secretary in the Christian Union, she arranged for Len to sing at one of their college outreaches. He was also Pastor of a large church in the South of England.

Well! It was love at first sight. From selling Len's gospel music in the local Christian bookshop, she became his wife! They married in July 1977 at Heather's church, Halford House in Richmond (just outside of London).

They pastored in England together, until moving to Australia in 1981. Len had been sent there by his mother as a small child, where he remained until returning to England at the age of 21. After his conversion, studying at Bible College and getting married, he felt a strong call to return to Australia. It wasn't so easy for Heather, but she willingly (albeit painfully) left her father and mother, sisters and lifelong friends, to travel across the world with her husband. They arrived in Australia with their 18-month old son Matthew, ready to start a completely new life. Their only daughter, Hannah was born during the following year, and so their young family was complete.

Len and Heather have now been in ministry together for 40 years. Len pastors the church, preaching and teaching God's Word. Heather leads the worship team, writes some of the worship songs they sing, plays keyboard in the band, and preaches every now and again. They live on the Gold Coast in Queensland, Australia, in one of the most beautiful parts of the most spectacular countries in the world.

(Well, someone has to!)